Never Knew I Needed:

The Story of Nanny Jean, Dementia Nan, and Me

Based on the blog:

Livingwithdementiablog.wordpress.com

I0412555

By Kirsty Elgar

With Nanny Jean's express permission

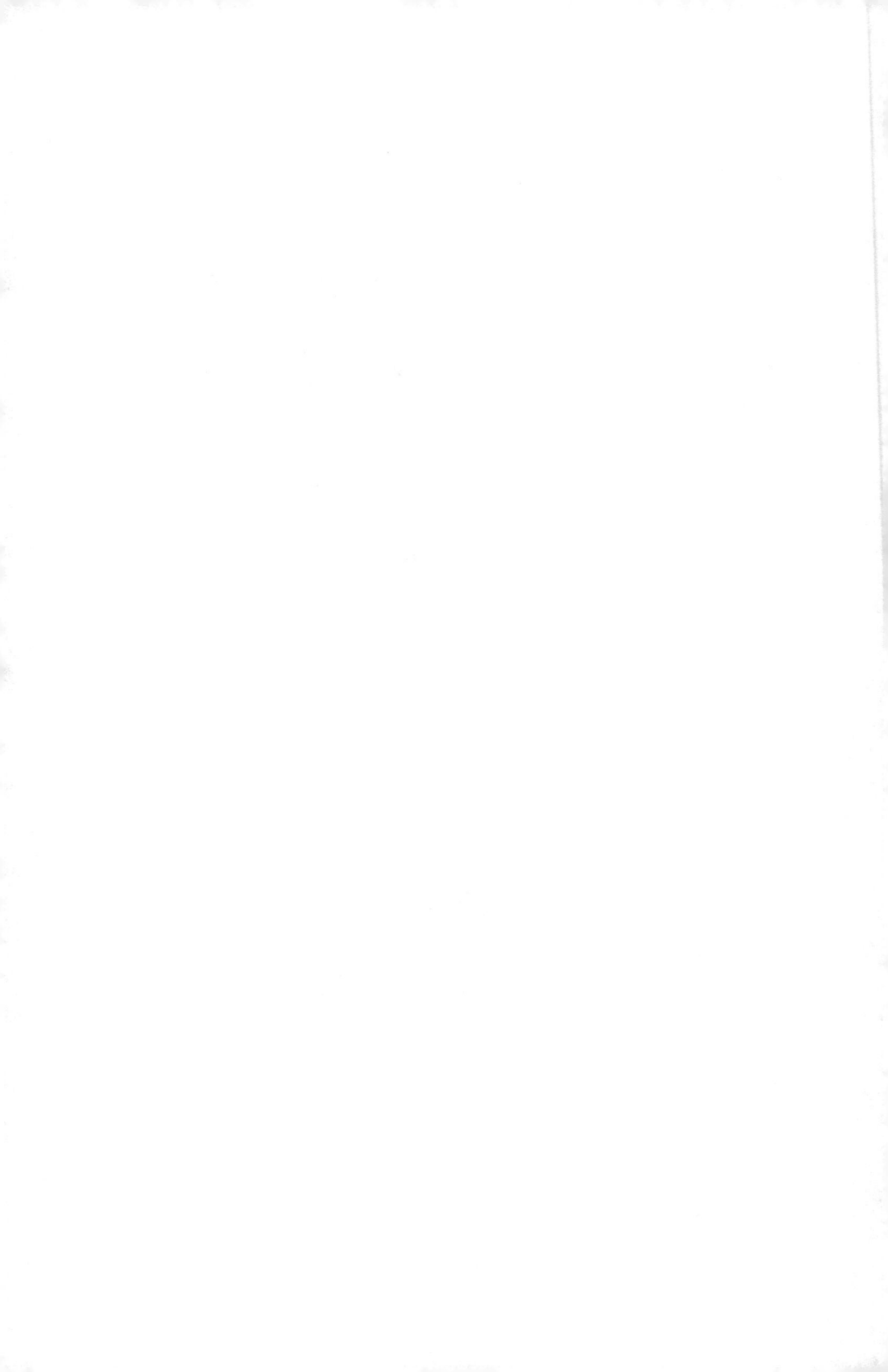

Dedication:

This is of course dedicated to Nanny Jean, without whom I would have had nothing to write about.

"You'll remember me, the one that can't remember"

Nanny Jean, Feb 2014

Table of Contents

Acknowledgements:

I have an obscene amount of people that I would like to thank. From the people directly involved in the writing process, to the people who supported the blog, to the people who have helped shape the person I have become. There is an extended list on my blog as I couldn't possibly name everybody here.

Firstly to my Nan, Nanny Jean – I am so grateful to be allowed to write so intimately about your life, and to be encouraged by you to share it with the world really is a blessing.

To my family – Thank you for putting up with me when I was at my worst, and for pushing me so hard to be my best.

Jennie – My Admiral Nurse. For all your support, teachings and encouragement I will be forever in your debt.

To my closest friends; Abi, Amy, the Ohana, Laura, Marc, and Team Casey's – Every one of you has had an impact on me, and helped me become who I am. Thank you for being my shoulders to cry on, life advisors, love gurus, and genuinely the best people a girl could wish for.

To everyone who has supported Nanny Jean and I through social media; from the bottom of my heart, thank you for encouraging us to keep plodding on. My absolute heartfelt thank you to anybody who purchases this book. You've made my dream come true.

Introduction:

The chapters are split into "information" and "diary entries". These are marked in the Contents so if you wish to read the diary parts before the information or vice versa it should be pretty simple to navigate.

N.B "caree" is a term coined by the Twitter community I spoke to, a nicer and easier word to use than "patient" or "sufferer" as Nanny Jean is so much more to me than a patient, as are the people I cared for professionally. And I still reject the idea that people "suffer" from dementia, hopefully my book will help you see there is a life after diagnosis that is not as bleak as the media portray.

N.B I always felt guilty when I moaned, so I found it easier to metaphorically split my Nan into two parts. Nanny Jean is my caring, funny, generous relative. Dementia Nan is the occasionally spiteful lady that I struggled to handle. Sometimes it really was best just to get it off my chest, and by detaching the dementia from my Nan it helped me to ease the guilt.

Preface:

In July 2012 I moved in with my Nan, also known as Nanny Jean, to help her around the house after a series of falls. I'll admit, I had selfish reasons too. I needed a place to live in order to save up and go travelling. But it turned out to be an arrangement that helped us both in ways that we were not expecting.

After a short while of living with Nan I began to notice differences in her behaviours and actions. My family and I delved into research and spoke with doctors, who could not initially give a formal diagnosis as Nanny Jean refused to have a memory test.

One reason she has since given for this refusal, is the stigma attached to memory problems. That older people should just learn to accept cognitive deterioration as a part of getting old. As well as the misconceptions that surround mental illness.

We were all certain it was a form of dementia. I started to do more for her around the house, and as her dementia worsened I picked up any slack and tried to help her emotionally. (We have since had an official diagnosis of mixed dementia with Lewy Body, thought to be caused by a series of mini strokes – there is more information on my blog of the various forms of dementia, their possible causes and effects).

It didn't take long for it to start to affect me mentally, and, after what seemed like 100 comments from Nanny Jean that I should write a book about all the "barmy" (her word, not mine) things she does, I started the blog. After each post I would give Nanny Jean the bare bones of what I had written and check she was OK with it. I'm not sure if she only said yes because she didn't understand what I was talking about, but she had great moments of clarity. She told me that as long as I tell the truth, and it helps somebody understand, she doesn't mind what I write.

I have kept Nan continuously updated of progress with the blog, she is astounded that so many people have wanted to hear about her life. And in so many different parts of the world (to date 19,000 people in 90 countries). She told me that not a lot of people can do what I do. I don't have the heart to tell her that the internet is full of people like me.

I had originally intended for the blog to be a viewing point for my friends and family to see what I was dealing with behind the scenes. But it did so much more, it gave me an outlet, explained to relatives why my emotions were all over the place, connected me with strangers who validated my feelings, understood and shared experiences, and above all it helped me show so many people what is like living with dementia, not just from the perspective of the person diagnosed, but from those who are closest to them. It is so much more than memory loss.

I realise of course that I am not the only person in this situation but I want people to know that they are not alone. I want to keep on raising awareness as people still find dementia something to joke about (-I will touch on comedy later as I do think it can be a great coping mechanism if used in the right way).

There are certain misconceptions attached to dementia that make it hurtful to joke about, for the caree and their friends and family.

To have the opportunity to turn my little blog into a book is incredible, I hope to share my experiences with so many other people, give you all a talking point, make dementia less taboo, and a little easier to understand.

And hopefully help you see that it doesn't have to be all darkness and sorrow. Living with and caring for my Nan has helped me in ways I could never have imagined.

Ultimately I wish to help people live with dementia, not suffer from it.

Chapter 1:

February 2013:

"Today I experienced my first big drama in caring for Nanny Jean. I think we've done well to have experienced no incidents before this. Anyway, I spent the morning reading in my room, and left Nanny Jean to potter, just like any other day. Except, I thought, something smells funny. I wandered downstairs, where the smell of acrid burning hit my nose. Following the smoke I ran to the kitchen to find the remains of a boiled dishcloth. I am unsure why the dishcloth was in a saucepan to begin with. Is this something all older people do? Or is it a Nanny Jean thing? Was she planning dishcloth soup for lunch? Answers on a postcard please.

Nanny Jean hadn't noticed the smell, had forgotten she was a boiling a dishcloth, couldn't remember putting it on in the first place and she certainly doesn't have the agility to sprint into action should anything further had happened. Needless to say I replaced the smoke alarms and have decided to keep a bit of a closer eye on my nanna."

This was my first sign that Nan would require additional support, and that potentially something deeper was going on as opposed to the effects of growing old. I spent months worrying that if I left the house she would set herself on fire and not be able to get out of the house. I ended up wrapping both of us in cotton wool which turned out to be the worst thing for both of us.

*   *   *

"Today we had the social services round, something I had been worrying and stressing about as Nanny Jean can be pretty vocal about her distrust and disliking of them. I think she worries that they will cart her off and put her in a care home against her will. But there was nothing to worry about, as would become a habit for Nanny Jean she proved me wrong. She and the social lady bonded right away over a mutual love of cheese sandwiches and Drambuie.

It was agreed that we both need a little extra support but Nanny Jean can stay in her own home as long as we have someone to keep an eye out for her (this is mostly for my own sanity and my mum's peace of mind)."

I don't know why I ever worried about things like the social worker visits. In the end they did nothing but help us and listened to my own and Nan's wishes which enabled us to keep her safe and comfortable in her own house for many years. Nanny Jean even grew to accept, appreciate and love the new people in her life who were initially there to help her physically, but who also stopped her from getting lonely and bored. They gave her the emotional support that I wasn't always equipped to give.

The Little Things:

"The funny thing about caring for Nan is how much it is opening my eyes to my own behaviour and thought process. My main struggle is how to deal with things. The bigger problems and issues I can cope well enough with, it really is the little things that put me on the edge of a breakdown.

These little things have no immediate risk, nothing that would put Nanny Jean in danger. But living with minor irritations such as repetitive conversations (especially about the weather, or impending night time), multiple losses of the same object or finding said object in an unusual location, 24 hours a day, seven days a week, can turn them into infuriating disputes. Which in turn just causes more problems for Nanny Jean, Dementia Nan and I."

Looking back I know all of the little things that drove me barmy seem petty; like the sound of a certain television presenter's voice, looking for the same object multiple times daily, and answering the same question every five minutes. But being thrown headfirst into Dementia Nan's reality time (this was the amount of time she would remain "lucid" and lasted around twenty minutes at the onset of the dementia) on repeat all day, every day, with no professional support, no one that really understood the situation and no previous experience to compare it to, made me feel like my head would combust.

My main "little thing", the one big grumble I really struggled to cope with was...the central heating. (Honestly, it was such a big little problem for so long I feel like it deserves a bigger build up, with dramatic music).

This was the main cause of most of the arguments in our household, the bone of contention between us. Nanny Jean was always cold, I was always too hot. I worried about the cost of having the heating on too much, Dementia Nan had no concept of money. Of course after a while I learned the golden rule of caring for someone living with dementia.

NEVER ARGUE WITH THE ACTIONS OF A PERSON WITH DEMENTIA.

Assume the caree is always right, and go with the flow. Besides things tend to work out better for everyone when we are all on the same side. This was taught to me by my Admiral Nurse Jennie (more on her later).

The following excerpt from my blog demonstrates one example of the stress I put myself through over the central heating;

"We had worked out a system that was working, by using a timer, so that the heating comes on while we sleep, and the house stays warm. However I had an early night, Dementia Nan turned the heating off completely. And we both woke up cold and grumpy. When I came downstairs I discovered that Dementia Nan had turned our gas oven on to heat the house, completely unaware of the potential dangers (apparently heating the house with the oven is another one of those things that older people used to do – like boiling dishcloths, but I'm not convinced). I turned the oven off and told her that I would

appreciate her not burning the house down this early in the morning. Predictably we soon had a cross Nanny Jean and a cross granddaughter."

I'm unsure why she insisted on turning it off so regularly, as sometimes it would be an accident, her confusion making it difficult to know which way to turn the dial. And other times Nanny Jean would deliberately turn it off because she didn't like the little red light indicating that the heating was on. We still have this conversation about the plug behind the television and its own indicator light, she doesn't like going to bed knowing that anything is turned on. I can only assume this is because when she was younger electricity was not as safe.

Thankfully we soon made up, but the whole situation, as well as others, could have been avoided if I hadn't stressed so much about the little things. I will talk more about coping mechanisms later but I regret not paying more attention to the golden rules. Or not discovering them earlier in order to have lived more peacefully. The older I get the more I realise how little use stress and worrying have. Nothing gets done by stressing, except creating tension.

Admiral Nurse/Guardian Angel:

After about six months of being a full time carer for Nan with no real support I was put into contact with an Admiral Nurse. A Registered nurse with experience in dementias who helps not just the caree but the carer in any way they can, be it practical, clinical or emotional. My mum did some research and found Jennie after I chewed her ear off about what was stressing me out; Dementia Nan's triggers, how to help Nanny Jean and multiple other complications.

I don't know how long I would have been able to help Nanny Jean without Jennie's support. We met regularly in a coffee shop, to encourage me to get out more, and she helped me understand the science side of dementia, the different types and their effects, as well as giving me tips on how to cope better (more on that later).

Jennie also taught me about Nanny Jean's increasing withdrawal. The reason for this is that Nanny Jean will be feeling constantly anxious, worrying about slipping up or being caught out. Due to her upbringing and the history of medical treatments she believes that a person displaying similar symptoms to her own, or any mental health issue, would be locked up in a home or asylum against their will.

That was why I decided to carry on helping her as long as I could. I felt, that if it was safe for both of us that it was better in the long run for her to be in her own home. I believed that if we put Nanny Jean into a care home she would give up fighting. This has thankfully been proven false, after much deliberation it was decided that Nan would receive better care from professionals in a residential home, and I've never seen her happier. The dementia has progressed rapidly, but she is surrounded by friends every day and loves to socialise with them, something I never thought I'd see. I do believe that being constantly surrounded by familiar objects and settings helped to delay the progression of her dementia at the onset but it is only possible to delay dementia for so long.

The Silence:

When I wrote about this on my blog I started with saying that it was so far my least favourite part of it all. Several years on and that still rings true, I'm certain it will always remain one of the hardest parts to witness, alongside no longer being recognised, not even as a friend.

Some days Nanny Jean will not say anything, for hours. Nor will she watch television, read, or listen to the radio. She will just sit and stare blankly at a wall. Barely responding to touch or any attempt at communication.

Jennie told me that Nanny Jean will start doing this whenever she feels the dementia creeping up. It impairs her ability keep up with storylines, or conversations. So she takes herself away from any situation where these might occur. Again, it keeps her from "slipping up" and potentially embarrassing herself.

This is why it makes me saddest. She is hiding herself. She feels like she cannot escape from it and allows it to consume her. Which is why I have tried so hard over the course of the last few years to distract her as much as possible, and to teach her to laugh at potentially embarrassing situations.

There was a time Nanny Jean would make me go into another room while she took her tights off, nowadays she is far more relaxed and allows us to help. Part of it may be the dementia, lessening her inhibitions, but I like to believe that I have helped her overcome the need for The Silence and given her more confidence in embracing her quirks.

Chapter 2:

March 2013:

"Nanny Jean and I have been having a really good couple of weeks, partly thanks to Jennie the Admiral Nurse helping me with my coping techniques. But also Nanny Jean seems different. Almost better somehow. I'm not naïve enough to think that this means that she is cured. I've known from the beginning that this is impossible. There is no cure for dementia. I also know that dementia works in waves, she will seem like she is recovering for a while and then one day there will be a sudden drop. I expect it will get harder, for both of us.

But for now I'm concentrating on the positives. Nanny Jean is chirpy most days, we've been having some great conversations, just inane chat but real quality time. There have been no disasters. Nan has been asking more questions, trying to stay in the conversation and not drifting out of it. She has been eating, like really eating. I can always tell when Nan isn't feeling great, she completely loses her appetite and barely even touches pudding.

Nanny Jean seems to be more grateful too. Of course I don't expect it, but it feels remarkable, and can really change a rubbish week around, to every now and again receive a genuinely heartfelt thankyou (and the hugs that usually accompany the gratitude are more than welcome too)! Nan seems to be enjoying having a bit more freedom, she's helping me pick recipes for dinners, and always looking for something to do around the house to help out. This was something I always used to reject, I didn't want her to help. In my mind she was too fragile, too easily broken and I didn't want to risk anything happening to her. But of course she is not made of glass, and is perfectly capable of grating cheese, slicing mushrooms, washing up, and even ironing (just so long as someone is keeping an eye on her, and a nose out for burning).

I suppose that all of this is helping her confidence (more on this later), which is something she definitely lacked before. This confidence is making her happier, she doesn't feel like so much of a failure, which is making her feel more comfortable. All of which combine to make one much happier Nan, and an easier life for both of us."

The difference in Nanny Jean that I had noticed would have also been down to her picking up on my emotions. From my experience, people with dementia are much more in tune with the people around them, and any underlying feelings. She would have been feeding off of my anxiety and stress, which was eliminated after I changed my reactions to the situations and eased up on the pressure I was putting on myself to be perfect.

*　　　　　　　*　　　　　　　*

""Knock, Knock"

"Who's there?"

"Oh just a random stranger"

"Come in"

My main frustration this week. Not bad jokes, but Nanny Jean's disregard for her own safety. She will open the door and welcome absolutely anybody in, despite having had money stolen by a drop in caller just months ago. I know she can't help it, that it becomes routine and an automatic reflex to see who is behind the door, but I worry that she doesn't think about herself or the consequences.

All of the people that are meant to be coming to the house can let themselves in, such as the carers, doctors, hairdresser, so anyone knocking on the door is usually not welcome. I tried putting signs on the door for Nan to read, but they've been there so long now it is almost as if they have become part of the door, or see through. For all the good they are doing they may as well not be there.

This is something that is really driving me to my wits end (again, just the little things). How can I prevent her from opening the door to strangers without barricading her in? With me being home 24/7 at the moment I'm really beginning to notice the dangers and risks she exposes herself to, either through ignoring them or being unable to perceive them."

Of course Nanny Jean doesn't have a disregard for her own safety, the dementia just eliminates the idea of risk. And she doesn't remember being robbed, which is probably for the best as it shook me up for weeks. I'm glad she didn't have to suffer with the nerves and fright. And we have implemented a lot more security around and outside the house now.

The signs and notices on the door were a great idea for a while. But after a period of time the dementia part of Nans brain didn't register that they were any different to the rest of the door, it had become routine to have them there. There were also issues with Dementia Nan taking offence to the notes, they made her feel like she was unable to do anything without being criticised, and why shouldn't she open the door to her own house?

That's why part of me thought she was ignoring the dangers. There were times that she was so determined to prove to herself, and me, that she was able to carry on living without my help that she would expose herself to risk seemingly on purpose.

Routine/Topsy Turvy:

"As I'm sure many people will agree (myself included) the key to a better quality of life is having some kind of routine or structure. Get up, go to work, come home, eat dinner, relax, and go to bed. This is especially true for those with an illness affecting their brains and psychology, like dementia. The routine can help trigger memories, and keep people active and living independently (with a little support) for as long as possible. Muscle memory certainly lasts longer, which is why we tend not to forget how to ride a bicycle, or in Nanny Jean's case, how to knit.

It may sound silly but I have found that Nanny Jean bases her routine around what is on the television."

I suppose that this is because people living with dementia can lose their ability to read a clock, as well as any other aspect of time. So, basing a daily routine around television programming is a pretty steady way of gauging the day. It is fairly constant.

Nanny Jean can no longer tell the time by looking at a clock. It started with a struggle to read a traditional clock face, but it has progressed into the inability to read the numbers on an enlarged digital clock. It is not just the numbers, but the perception of time. If she is told the time of day she will not know if it is daytime or night time, which is leading to her wanting to go to bed earlier and earlier.

Telling the differences between times of day is not the only difficulty she faces. Nanny Jean has no grasp on which day, month, season or even year it is. This is something that has developed with the worsening of the dementia. As yet it is causing no detrimental effects to her wellbeing so I'm learning not to stress about it, however this was quite challenging when I first moved in with Nan and was treated to several renditions of "it looks like rain" every time she closed the curtains at sundown. I gave up trying to explain that the sky was dark because night was falling and instead took it upon myself to close all curtains in the house just to avoid having that same conversation again.

Here is an example of Nanny Jean's day by television: breakfast with morning medication before the feuding families. Housework and laundry during the daily magazine shows. Lunch is served at half past twelve on the dot. Tea and biscuits follow, during the antique or property programmes. Then it is time to sit, chill and chat during the quiz shows. When the evening news starts it is time to ask Nanny Jean what she would like for dinner. This is because it is set in her routine to always have dinner at the start of the evening soaps. (This was the case even when I was a child and stayed with her and my granddad for a holiday). I keep her updated with the storylines while the soaps are on, and once the night time news starts it is time for bed.

"So imagine the trouble I was in on one particular Thursday when dinner came to Nanny Jean halfway through her first soap, which had started fifteen minutes early. Our evening only got worse as the soap was an hour long special, and led to Nanny Jean missing half of another soap on a different channel. This left her more confused than usual about who the characters were, what they were

doing and why. I honestly find it hard enough to follow the plotlines as it is, so trying to explain the first half of a television programme that I hadn't seen was darn near impossible. Especially for Nanny Jean to comprehend, as she then forgot the first thing I'd said as soon as I started a new topic."

I learned to overcome this eventually by memorising the blurbs in the television programming magazine for each day. Any questions about the plot would be answered with a quick two sentence summary of the soap for the day.

"And don't get me started on the complications of having the football on instead of the soaps. That throws Nanny Jean so out of whack that her whole evening is ruined."

At the time I wished that it was possible to put football on its own channel, and to keep regular television programming as regular as possible. I see now that that may be unreasonable. And there are so many ways we could have avoided any issues.

Firstly, I needn't have stressed about keeping Nanny Jean completely informed about the missed storylines. I knew she would forget them anyway. She wouldn't lose sleep over it. I could have made anything up (and probably come quite close to a storyline from at least one of the soaps), this would have kept her happy and prevented a cross Dementia Nan from making evenings more difficult for both of us.

Secondly, I could have recorded some soaps from across the week and put those on while football was playing. Or I could have just not stressed about it and found a distraction, like Jennie the Admiral Nurse would have recommended. These blips in our routine were never regular occurrences, and it does people good to be spontaneous every now and again. Would it have hurt to play some games, watch a film or sort through photographs? Looking back I was so hell bent on ensuring Nanny Jean continued to live her regular life that I was finding it hard to make any allowances to our routine. Changes that could in fact have benefitted her.

Chapter 3:

April 2013:

"Yesterday we learned of the death of Baroness Thatcher. I was hoping that this would invoke some more talk about dementia, but the news coverage so far has seemed to skim over the fact that she had been diagnosed with it. This topic has given me a great deal to think about so apologies if this post is a little higgledy piggledy.

Firstly, I wanted to elaborate on something I said on social media yesterday, 140 characters just isn't enough to convey my feelings eloquently. I understand that some people have been, possibly still are, deeply affected by policies that were implemented during Thatcher's time as Prime Minister. But I have heard some truly vile things being said in the last twenty four hours. And I'm struggling to find a defence for them. It is bad enough to be disrespectful about the dead, organising street parties to celebrate her death when her poor family are mourning?! I can't describe how angry and sick that makes me feel. But to me it feels so much more hateful and harsh, knowing that Lady Thatcher had dementia.

The lady who died yesterday would have been a shadow of the former Baroness, and it could even be said that the Prime Ministerial Thatcher died around the time of the onset of her dementia.

The second thought that was prompted by the death of Lady Thatcher was about how anybody can get dementia. It is not something anyone can avoid, or even cure, no matter how rich and powerful they are,

17

or used to be. And this has only been proven time and time again with multiple well known personalities being diagnosed with dementia.

My final thought for the day, is something I would like to publicly voice. I am so disappointed with the media, who could have seized this opportunity to raise awareness of dementia, carers, charities and support networks. But they have almost managed to ignore it completely, some hardly even acknowledging that Margaret Thatcher had dementia. Instead, they fuel the public hatred and focus on the negativity that this event has brought out in some of the nation's people, giving them coverage they most certainly do not deserve, or need."

In hindsight I regret the phrasing that made it sound like Thatcher died when she developed dementia, or that she became a shadow of herself. It is something that I learned, when I was caring for Nan, is not necessarily true. With the right care and attention dementia does not have to completely eradicate a person. And something I positively advocate now is that there is life after a diagnosis of dementia.

Dementia is becoming more and more prevalent, diagnoses are occurring more and more frequently, and yet people still view it as something that "won't happen to me". But it can happen to anybody, and more needs to be done to stop people sweeping it under the rug. By talking about it we can aid public awareness leading to faster and better diagnoses, more support for carees and those closest to them, and better funding for research and care.

We are in need of better support as there is currently no way to stop dementia. It is fatal.

Activities/Whistle While You Work:

"Dementia is now part of your relationship with your loved one, learn how to cope with, deal with, and live with it" – Dementia workshop, Home Instead

In the last chapter I mentioned that doing some activities may have distracted Nanny Jean from her (and my) issues with the television. I was lucky enough to attend a dementia workshop in the summer after I started caring for Nan. (I ended up being employed by the company who were running the workshop and working as a carer specialising in dementias). And they really brought home for me how important the use of activities can be for someone living with dementia, or even the person caring for them.

Obviously activities are beneficial to us all, they give us stimulation, as well as a sense of purpose and accomplishment (I certainly feel like I have done something worthwhile with my day if I manage to hoover). So for people like Nanny Jean, who are living dementia, this is even more important. Remembering what Jennie the Admiral Nurse had said about the dementia making Nan feel constantly anxious, surely if she completes an activity it will ease that feeling.

For people living with dementia doing an activity can also help to decrease the likelihood of potentially damaging behaviours such as wandering or aggression, by reducing boredom and depression.

And it's not just the science side. From my experiences with Nanny Jean I can confirm how much more fun the atmosphere becomes if both the carer and caree are able to have a laugh whilst participating in activities. It also gives the carer better memories of their loved one, dementia does not have to be about watching a person slip away. Personally some of my best memories of Nanny Jean have been from the years I spent caring for and living with her.

There are three different types of activities:

* Activities that stimulate the mind

* Activities that exercise the body

* Activities that encourage social interaction

It is important to encourage activities that work on improving all three areas. Physical fitness is important to build muscle memory and strength, to reduce the risk of falls. Social interaction and mental stimulation are important for increasing emotional wellbeing, which in turn will build the comfort of the caree.

It is also important to remember any limitations and preferences of the caree. For example Nanny Jean is as much of a social hermit as me, and prefers one on one interaction as opposed to being part of a group.

Activities don't have to be fancy or elaborate, something as simple as encouraging Nanny Jean to help with household chores helped to build her confidence, physical fitness and hand to eye co-ordination. She loves to help out with dusting, as soon as she sees me undertaking any housework she wants to join in. Other people may require more prompting, but inclusion is always flattering, just give them the option. (Tips on how to encourage the less enthusiastic can be found in the next chapter). And of course with Nanny Jean helping out my own chores became less taxing and I had more time to "relax".

There are more detailed ideas for activities on my blog site but one of my favourite personalised activities that Nanny Jean and I did together was creating her life book. It is a scrap book about Nanny Jean's life with photographs and notes, as well as any other sorts of prompts and triggers for memories and conversations. It includes old sweet wrappers, fabric from old clothes, and an old cat collar. We found it especially useful when introducing external care to encourage one on one interaction. We also use the life book to find ways to distract Dementia Nan and bring Nanny Jean back.

Getting Nanny Jean to do something physical was hard. We were both paranoid after her series of falls, and as such she never used to get up out of her chair much for fear of falling. (It is important to consult with a doctor before starting any physical activity as it may aggravate existing conditions).

I found a website that contains exercises suitable for older people (some of them I found to be a little ambitious and out of both Nanny Jean's and my own ability range). But I think the stretching was beneficial to her. Nowadays she gets up and potters round the house periodically throughout the day so I know she is keeping mobile. While Nanny Jean does her gentle stretches I do my slightly more energetic workouts with some music going. It makes Nan laugh to see how puffed out and sweaty I get while she sits in her chair and does arm raises.

Mentally stimulating Nanny Jean was initially done by playing various board games, cards, puzzles and crossword books, but as her sight deteriorated these became less viable options. We had been encouraged after one of Nan's visits to hospital to help her eat more balanced meals. If left to her own devices Nanny Jean was prone to living off egg and chips, or cheese on toast.

To avoid her missing out on vital nutrients and to help stimulate her mental processes I got her involved with planning and preparing dinners. I think her favourite task was grating the cheese, as I always caught her sneaking chunks of cheese to nibble when she thought I wasn't looking.

We also encouraged her to choose her own lunches from the meals on wheels service. Unfortunately she had a habit of ordering meals that she didn't like. For example, one day she had chicken and mushroom pie delivered. But she told me she doesn't like pie, or mushrooms. (This was the first I had heard of it, as we often have mushrooms to bulk out evening meals and I can guarantee if I serve chicken pie tonight she would eat the whole thing, except the crust. I always burn the crust). So she ate her mash, picked out the vegetables (Nanny Jean would never eat a vegetable by choice, no matter how much emotional blackmail is involved) and wolfed down her pudding. I have found a way to sneak the leftover vegetables from lunch into her evening meals, and as yet she doesn't seem to have noticed.

Giving Nan the choice, and tasks to do that help with preparing dinner is giving her more confidence, as well as encouraging muscle memory from stirring, slicing and grating.

In the many months that Nanny Jean and I have cooked together there has only been one meal that she openly told me she hadn't enjoyed (the others I'm assuming she enjoyed as there were no vocal complaints, or leftovers). Lasagne. Because, as she informed me halfway through eating it, she doesn't like pasta. I have found that the dementia has changed her eating habits too, bacon sandwiches used to be a staple; now she hates bacon and due to a diminished chewing and swallowing ability food has to be a lot mushier.

Chapter 4:

May 2013:

"Nanny Jean has been a lot chirpier since I have started implementing some of the techniques I learned from the dementia workshop. Except for today, I felt poorly so I spent most of the day asleep, and consequently Nan has spent most of the evening stropping as she had no one to talk to. I think she thought I was deliberately ignoring her.

Anyway, to update you with how our week has been. Last Saturday Nanny Jean had been complaining of lower back ache. This was nothing out of the ordinary, so I sorted her out with some medication and we carried on with the rest of our day with no problems. By the evening Nan was wincing and told me the pain had spread to her neck, Nanny Jean has never been one to voice her discomfort so this concerned me. And when she mentioned her pain to my mum on the evening phone call I was prompted into action.

I have to admit that I had been putting off involving the doctor or other medical professional, for fear that they would recommend she went into hospital. Nanny Jean detests hospitals and I didn't want her to blame and resent me if she ended up there. This wasn't great logic on my part, thinking back on it. If I hadn't called the doctor she may have got sicker and would have definitely gone to hospital, and may have even had to stay there longer!

So I called the out of hour's doctor, having completely forgotten that they don't have out of hours' anymore. Instead I had to call the non-emergency-emergency number 111. I'm certain the girl who answered was a new trainee as I could almost hear her following the flow chart of symptoms. I told her that my thoughts and concerns were for my Nan's kidneys, as they have caused her problems before. We ran through Nanny Jean's temperature, she was cold. And then...RED ALERT!!! The girl told me she was going to have to call an ambulance as it could be Nan's heart. (I know I'm not a qualified doctor but I'm pretty sure that even with dementia playing tricks on her mind my Nan can tell the difference between her heart and lower back). We were then informed that the girl could not find the number for an ambulance... (?!) And we were prompted to call 999. Oh wait, never mind, the girl has found the number. The ambulance will be with us in 8 minutes, could we please be ready to go?"

As a side note I would like to point out that I am not complaining, this girl may well have been new to the job and she was very friendly and helpful. It all just felt a little dramatic.

"A long 8 minutes later (I didn't time them, but I know for certain it was less than half an hour – which is a much better wait time than we have experienced in the past) the ambulance people arrived, clearly expecting a heart attack victim. Still, they checked Nanny Jean over, agreed it could be her kidneys and told her she would have to go with them to the hospital. I was expecting a lot of drama, after all Nan had become very stressed with the waiting and the pain and the drama but I was pleasantly surprised. My praise for the paramedics really kicks

in here. I mentioned to them before they entered the house that Nan has dementia so a little more care is required. And they were perfect, obviously Nan told them there was no need for a hospital and tried to refuse, but they somehow managed to convince her it was a good idea. (They must have Jedi mind powers). They did a few more checks in the ambulance and rushed her straight into a ward as soon as we arrived at the hospital.

For the first five minutes maybe, Nan was fine. Very well behaved, very polite. Then she got impatient, and a bit naughty." (Naughty Nan is my favourite, she gets very cheeky and likes to test people's limits. As long as it isn't my limits being tested I find it very entertaining). *"She started singing "why are we waiting". Asking me in a louder voice than I thought she possessed if we were waiting for Christmas. And when could we go home? When I told my mum about Nanny Jean's naughtiness she told me that it must be my effect on Nan, as whenever my mum has had to take her to the hospital, or even a doctor's surgery, she gets very quiet and reserved. Oops.*

Instead of the hospital writing us off as a paranoid relative and over dramatic elderly person (which for some reason I was expecting, see my later chapter on misconceptions) they checked everything thoroughly; ECG, bloods, urine, everything. And not until every result had come back clear would they let us go. The staff regularly came to check on Nan, despite how busy they were and how naughty she was, and made sure she had what she needed. They even offered an extra blanket when she said she was cold.

They were gentle when taking her bloods, or making her more comfortable in the bed.

All in all we were at the hospital just over two hours, we weren't left on a bed in a corridor. The whole place was clean. I saw each nurse wash her hands about a million times. And I left with nothing bad to say about the NHS, as well as peace of mind that there were no underlying issues with Nan. I'd like to take this opportunity to thank the nurses and doctors who were involved with Nan that night, especially the paramedics who comforted her, she couldn't speak highly enough of you while we were waiting.

The following morning Nan told me she had enjoyed her trip out. Which makes me glad that she may no longer be as nervous of going to hospital. But also a little concerned that she may now try to go more frequently as it was so enjoyable."

Thankfully Nanny Jean hasn't felt a need to call the paramedics back, and has been relatively healthy. She has had the odd fall, and many in call visits from the doctor but no need to rush off to a hospital for the moment. Of course thanks to the dementia she has no idea she even visited a hospital last year, let alone that three years ago she spent most of the year in hospital after falling so frequently. I am thankful in a way that she doesn't remember as it means she isn't as worried. But it concerns me that most of the time she is unaware of her physical limitations. The nurses believed however that this in fact aided her recovery process after breaking her hip. Her body forgot that it was broken and allowed to rehabilitate much more quickly. Either that or she's superhuman.

Involvement/Involve Me and I Learn:

I'm hoping that in this part of the chapter I can cover how to encourage involvement in some of the previously mentioned activities as well as others which can be found listed on my blog.

It is important to stimulate all of the senses, any one of them could hold the trigger to a memory or emotion. Here are examples of how to use the senses to help a person living with dementia;

* Touch – A person living with dementia may not be able to recognise when they are being spoken to, but a small squeeze of their hand, or stroking their arm will reassure them of a familiar presence and their involvement. Different textures can also be used to stimulate the brain (I will cover this in more detail in the Montessori chapter).

* Hearing – I have found music to be especially helpful. I often have music on around the house which I know Nanny Jean knows from her past, or sing while I'm cooking and cleaning. On a good day Nan will be able to name the band or song; "Perhaps" is a particular favourite, or "Boogie Woogie Bugle Boy". However if I'm really lucky there have been occasions where Nan will join in singing! We have had some great renditions of "Consider Yourself" and "Singing in the Rain".

* Smell – Smells are often the strongest trigger for memories, for example the smell of my moisturizer brings back vivid memories of a holiday in Florida three years ago. When Nanny Jean found an old perfume hidden in the depths of a drawer and spritzed it, it brought back memories of all the times

she had worn it. It had been her personal favourite when she had been working in London so I was treated to stories about what it was like in the capital many years ago.

* Taste – By communicating with someone and listening to them or looking out for non-verbal triggers it is possible to find out information about their favourite meals, either from their childhood, or a special occasion that they attended. By cooking meals that they enjoyed in their past there is a chance to help trigger a memory and to create a new one.

* Sight – Something as simple as seeing the family pet, or a photograph from long ago can trigger a memory and a story. If this is not working I have found that using a variety of colours can help to comfort and relax Nanny Jean and delay any potential anxiety. Nan loves flowers, so my mum often gets bouquets delivered "just because". Seeing the gift makes my Nan feel appreciated, and when she notices them on the sideboard it gives her an activity to do, as she prunes and cares for them, and obviously spends time smelling each flower, but this only has any effect with the more potent ones.

The easiest ways to encourage a person living with dementia to get involved with activities are to:

* Offer simple choices, and drip feed information.

Don't bombard them with all the information at once as it becomes overwhelming and they become defensive. For example Nanny Jean detests the idea of having a bath (once she gets in there she loves it, but it is the task of getting her to the bathroom that has always been a challenge). So now I ask her:

* Now OR Later?

* Bath OR Shower?

This way I am still giving her the choice and an ability to make a decision, but it is harder for her to refuse or argue. There is no option or trigger for not having a bath so it cancels that option in her brain.

* Start without them.

People don't like to be left out, if a caree knows that there is an opportunity to join in they will probably want to, especially if the carer looks like they're having fun (I find this hard when washing up, it is the bane of my life).

* Offer encouragement. NEVER CRITICISE.

I think one of the biggest and most important lessons that I have learned while caring for Nan would be that to question anything a person living with dementia is doing, is to question their thoughts, mind set and leads to destructive behaviour. Everyone is much happier and more comfortable when reading from the same page. It is impossible to reason with a person with dementia, so what is the harm in joining their way of thinking? (As long as there is no risk of danger for any party).

* Ask them for help.

I have found that Nanny Jean is a lot more herself (and less Dementia Nan) when she thinks that what she is doing is helping me or my mum. It's a nice feeling to do a favour for somebody and that is still a feeling that she is able to recognise.

Sometimes though there is no way around it, a foot will go down and Nanny Jean will not want to participate in anything I have planned. And I have come to learn that this is OK. Rather than stress both myself and Nan out by relentlessly badgering on about one thing it is much better for me to admit defeat and do something else. Besides, a quiet lazy day is always better than a day of chores anyway.

One thing that bothers me is the idea of Nan watching television in a separate room with no interaction while I'm cleaning. I have found that bribery can also work as an incentive to join me, as demonstrated in this extract:

"Today I did the ironing, and to prevent Nan watching television in the other room, I made her a cup of tea (which is something she can never refuse) and set a newspaper on the table opposite me. Sure enough she came and sat with me, drinking her tea and chatting about articles she was finding in the paper. I can ask her until I'm blue in the face if she would like to join me while I'm in a different room of the house, but bribe her there with a cup of tea and there was no stress at all! It was nice to see her doing something different to looking at the television, even something as small as changing her surroundings and doing a different activity was

enough to see a difference in her attitude and behaviour".

Chapter 5:

June 2013:

"Had a gorgeous weekend with my mum in Somerset, my first time away from Nanny Jean since I moved in, and I'm only just getting back into a routine. As many topics as I still have on my list to cover I thought I should share with you all my feelings about the time away.

In a brief sentence, my weekend away made me feel like an over protective, over bearing parent.

Before I had even left London I had called Nan three times to check she was OK. I called her again when I got to Somerset to discover that she thought the carer had not fed the rabbit, so she had gone outside and done it herself. Nanny Jean ended up getting quite distressed because I could not stop myself asking questions about what the carer had done, and in the end my mum had to intervene and tell me to stop. This phone call left me feeling even guiltier about leaving Nan so I spent the rest of the evening being sad and with my heart racing from the stress of worrying about the what ifs.

Mum and I had a lovely morning the next day exploring the sights of Somerset and the Exmoor National Park. When we got home for lunch mum decided to call Nan. When Nan answered we could hear voices in the background and Nan could not or would not tell us who they were. We called the estate agents, neither of whom had arranged a viewing. So the panic set in again. Our lovely estate agent legged it down to the house to check Nanny Jean was OK, and told her off for letting people into the house, despite the now numerous signs on the door, and notes that I had left. She also left her phone number and insisted that if people do want entry to the house Nan should check with her. (Not that Nan would remember to do this, but the thought was nice). All the while mum and I were in a right tizz!

We later found out that the viewers were scheduled to have arrived that morning, and had decided that as they were late they would do it on their own. My mind was slightly eased except for the fact that I could now add worrying about who Nan is letting into the house on top of the worrying about medications, back pain, eating, cooking and possible fires, falling inside, falling outside and getting stuck there for the night...(And people wonder why I never go out).

So apart from the mishaps and my overactive worrying brain I had a great weekend. And found our future bungalow for Nan to move into while she still has the mental capacity to make that decision. (The idea of living this close to the seaside, fudge shops and Exmoor National Park helped her make her decision very quickly).

When I got home I checked through the carers' book, and it turns out that the letter I left for the carer had mysteriously disappeared. The letter outlining what needed doing to help Nan while I was away and asking them if they could feed the rabbit. I have my own theory about the letter, which I'm sure many of you can guess. I believe Nan may have read the letter, decided she could do it all herself and threw it away. Still as ferociously independent as *ever. And proving to me that despite all my fears and worries she is able to cope for a weekend without my 24/7 surveillance/care, just so long as I can bolt the door shut!"*

I still find it hard to leave Nan, and spend a lot of time when I'm away from her thinking about what she is doing and if she could be endangering herself. This is completely irrational, the amount of visits my Nan now has from carers, my mum and my sister amount to what I'm fairly certain is still 24 hour care. But is natural for someone who has ever been a carer.

It becomes an instinct to worry, and it is hard to let someone else take over that part of life, for however long or short a period of time. We all have that ingrained feeling that no one could do something as well as we have, especially as we are the only ones with the experience. And yet despite a few minor (and they really are minor in the grand scheme of things) mishaps I have found that the people we employ to help with Nanny Jean really know and love what they're doing and I am much more relaxed about handing some of Nan's care over to them.

Managing Behaviours/Be Prepared

An eventual problem for people living with dementia is the struggle to speak or write, to voice opinions or concerns. This struggle is what can lead to the internal anxiety and aggression that are linked to the external behaviours relating to the various types and stages of dementia.

The behaviours that can be associated with dementia (It should be noted that not everybody with dementia will display all, if any of these behaviours-dementia will affect every person differently):

* Delusions – truly believing they can see something, or have done something, that may not be true.

* Wandering

* Refusal - which can lead to physical aggression

* Repetition

* Agitation

* Sexual Inappropriateness

* False Accusations

Sometimes these behaviours will be easier than others to manage, and most of the time they will not require any action. Thinking of the golden rule again:

IF IT ISN'T HURTING ANYBODY DON'T POINT IT OUT/DON'T ARGUE ABOUT IT

In my experience, Nanny Jean and I are happier when we both accept her new world and I join her in it, rather than trying to drag her back to the "real" world.

Of course, if there had been any behaviour that could have been detrimental to her wellbeing then I would have done something to prevent harm. Harmful behaviours can be anything from;

* Refusing to eat/drink (Nanny Jean insists she is not hungry most of the time, but will eat about seven desserts in a row. And who can blame her, I'd love to eat seven desserts in a row)!

* Not frequently washing

* Refusing medication

* Striking out

* Withdrawing

It was possible, once I had been living with Nanny Jean for a few months to get to recognise the build up to any destructive behaviours. Mostly it was based on anxiety and stress. Again, the best preventative method was distraction. This has worked best for us when I need to coax Nanny Jean back out from Dementia Nan's dark cloud. This can be talking, about the weather is the easiest topic to catch Nan's attention, but also talking to her about the cat, my latest plans for world domination or what she fancies for dinner later. But I also use tea and biscuits, putting laundry away, dusting, anything to stop her thinking about what might be stressing her out.

If the distraction method isn't working then Nanny Jean is usually having trouble with communicating. When I suspect this is the problem I use prompting by asking what she needs and giving simple options for responses (more often than not it is trying to find a misplaced object, but can be a toileting need, hunger or pain).

Another thing I learned, from experience with Nan and other carees along with the workshop and training was:

DON'T RESPOND TO BAD BEHAVIOURS

If a person with dementia becomes angry, inappropriate or physical the best idea is to find a safe zone away from the caree. Reacting to bad behaviours gives the mind more exposure to the interaction, and a chance to create a new memory. This could encourage the belief that the caree will receive attention by throwing a walking stick or trying to kiss their carer (this has happened – more than once, not with Nanny Jean but a gentleman who I made house calls to with the care company. It took a firm reminder that his wife was in the next room and a quickstep to the side to avoid any damage being done).

Physical violence can be damaging not just to the caree, but also to the people around them. If a caree starts lashing out there is a chance that their carer could become injured. In this case there is no one to call for help or to reassure and comfort the caree. To escape the situation leaves two outcomes; that the caree injures themselves or the behaviour/attitude melts away and is forgotten.

Chances are with no one to witness their behaviour they will calm down pretty quickly, but if not then at least the carer is safe to administer first aid and if necessary call for help.

As previously mentioned dementia is very personal and affects everybody differently, every behaviour and/or mood swing is different. What can help a caree like Nanny Jean one minute, may not work the next.

The best option is to have more than one trick or technique, three is the ideal number. By preparing three different ways to deter a behaviour or even encourage involvement, there are extra possibilities for success. For example asking whether Nanny Jean would like a bath or shower. A little while later asking whether now or later is better. Then finally asking her to pick a bubble bath to sample.

ALWAYS TRY TO REMAIN CALM

I know from experience it is easier said than done. But people with dementia have high perception of other people's emotions and will react to what they can feel.

Here are some ideas for techniques to implement when trying to diffuse a high tension situation with a person with dementia;

* Apologise or take blame for the situation – (This is the one I struggle with, it gets frustrating having to constantly be the bad guy but it is easier for me to forget apologising for something that I haven't done

than it is for Nanny Jean to accept that she may have failed or slipped up in some way)

* Similarly to encouraging an individual to participate in an activity, use the simple options technique – Give them control over when or how or where they will be doing something, but don't tell them they will be doing it. Leave that to be implied.

* Redirect – Offer a treat such as chocolate (or fish and chips in Nan's case, as long as I buy fish and chips when (I) have done something wrong then everything is forgiven and OK).

* Physically remove items that can be used as weapons, such as walking sticks. This seems harsh but it is only a temporary solution while the atmosphere is tense. Once the situation is calmed and the walking stick is no longer likely to be used a flying missile it should obviously be returned to the owner. I would also suggest trying to remove it discreetly, the items that people with dementia keep near their person are guarded closely and they can be very possessive and volatile should somebody try to take them away.

Of course it doesn't matter how prepared I am, or how much experience and training a person has, some days are going to be rubbish. Some days Nanny Jean will be completely uncooperative, will refuse anything, and may hit "The Silence" temporarily. As mentioned previously when these days occur it is best to concentrate more on some rest and relaxation instead of getting worked up trying to solve every problem that might be encountered. The following is an example of a bad day I was having, which ended up being a bad day for Nanny Jean;

"Been a very strange sort of day today. I hardly slept last night, as some of you may be aware I am having a bad reaction to a fair few gnat bites. And the fire coursing through my legs kept me up. Still, I got up this morning regardless, feeling very much in need of a lazy day and not much talking.

So I got the DVD's out and Nan and I watched old home videos of me as a baby. She was laughing all through them, and comparing me as a baby to me now. Apparently there has been no change...not sure if that's a compliment or not! We then watched Despicable Me. And Nan loved it. She kept telling me how clever it was, but other than that I was able to chill. She was laughing along with the jokes and smiled at the happy ending so I think she followed the story quite well. She can't remember watching a film now though, let alone what the story was.

This evening however Nan has seemed very distant and unable to keep up with conversation. She hardly talked through dinner, and during Who Wants to Be a Millionaire we usually like to give the silly answers. But when I answered one of the questions with a silly response she glared at me, then nodded and said "yes. Family Trees trace teachers" as if I was an idiot for doubting it.

Nan has had a great couple of weeks with her memory so I was expecting a drop soon. But it was still a bit of a shock. She seems to be like a rollercoaster, I get used to one lapse and a few days/weeks/months later she drops again, and I have to get used to a whole new Nan.

She seems OK now, still not talking much. But I shall just have to keep an eye on her the next few days and monitor what it is that's making her feel as if she needs to withdraw.

That's the thing with dementia, you can never get used to it. It is constantly changing and deepening. Adding more and more layers to a more and more confusing illness."

The dips still occur, I suppose with moving to France for seven months I was expecting to see a deterioration so I was not too shocked to see the developments when I returned. However my mum and sister noticed a drastic change when we returned from a three week holiday. Having spoken to the doctor the bigger dips are caused by TIA's, the smaller ones associated more directly to the progress of the dementia. I've stopped trying to get used to it now, just taking every day as it comes. As ever, some days are much better than others, and it's those days that I live for.

Chapter 6:

Montessori and Every Child A Talker

It has been mentioned many times over that managing the behaviours of a person with dementia can be quite similar to the methods of managing children. That is not to say that they should be treated like a child, quite the opposite in fact. They have most likely lead a completely independent life up until the dementia, and so to suddenly be treated like a child again is demeaning.

It is more the manner in which a person reacts to and intercepts that should be done as if for a child. Many carers for people with dementia find these methods easier, as they have already had children and the experience aides the caring process. Young carers such as myself are doing it the other way round, so I'm learning the struggle now but the experience I have with Nan should be beneficial to me should I ever want children in the future.

I used to work in nurseries with children from three months up until four years, and despite them not being specifically Montessori nurseries we did of course use some of her techniques and influence. And I've realised, I am subconsciously using them with Nanny Jean as well as the more recent ECAT (Every Child a Talker). I think it's important to try and encourage and stimulate the use of verbal communication for those people with dementia who still have the ability to, as it could possibly delay the day when it is made impossible.

Montessori believed three things are needed to achieve potential in children. Independence, Freedom, and Respect, these three ideas are also things which are beneficial to people with dementia (or indeed all human beings). And they can be achieved in a home setting through:

* Choices of activity (Give them simple options: maximum three) - Just to re iterate a point I have made several times, promote choices. Let the caree be aware of the validity of their decisions. For example if Nanny Jean particularly enjoys dinner I remind her that she chose it.

* Uninterrupted work time – I interpret this so that it is not just limited to learning or work, but any activity that a caree is undertaking. It helps them to keep focused by removing distractions, such as the television

* Learning from doing NOT listening – By learning things practically, by doing activities themselves, they are building memories and muscle memory. Besides a person with dementia will not hear a lecture, they'll zone out and hear "buzz buzz mumble, mumble". Which means that lecturing really is a waste of time for everybody.

Montessori also believed in having an environment that reflected the needs of children. Or in our case our carees. (I dislike comparing my Nan to a child, but the dementia behaviours are the ones I'm tackling here. The dementia is the child, so to speak). The environment should be:

* Constructed in a way that is in proportion to their needs e.g. Nan cannot get upstairs, so we constructed her a bedroom downstairs and later moved to a bungalow to aid her mobility and ensure there was no temptation for her to try and tackle the stairs.

* Be clean and attractive. There is no point expecting a person to join in activities in the kitchen for example, to help prepare dinner, if it is a mess and there is clutter everywhere. Eliminate visual noise.

* Make sure things are in order. Nan loves tea, so the tea cup next to the container with teabags next to the milk jug next to the kettle. And the mandatory biscuit tin.

* Have an environment that won't hinder movement. Exercise of any form is vital to keep a loved one mobile and will help build muscle and stimulate the brain.

* Once again, whatever activity they are doing, lower distraction by only have those materials out. It helps lower confusion.

I have tried to simplify ECAT in a way that keeps it useable in relation to dementia. Hopefully these methods can be used to stimulate conversation skills and prolong verbal communication:

• Talk TO the person NOT at them – Always give them a chance to respond or answer, no matter how long they need. Watch them for signs of understanding such as head movements before repeating or changing the topic.

- Spend an allotted time each day dedicated to just conversation. Turn the television off, remove any distractions and chat for however long the caree can stay connected for. Nan can talk for hours some days and barely 5 minutes the next. So activities really are caree lead.
- Repeat words or sounds the individual makes to confirm meaning.
- Share a book / newspaper / magazine / poem / song every day and get them to join in and offer opinions. Not only stimulating vocal chords but giving them a chance to think independently. Nan loves to give her opinion on current affairs during the news, it's our designated moaning time.

My 10 Commandments

I don't think that there is a set way to care for a person with dementia, as demonstrated in this book, every aspect really can vary. But I have compiled a list of my ten commandments, that if I were to do this again, I would pay more attention to.

1) Don't Argue! Do not scold, learn to go with the flow. As I have discussed trying to reason with an individual who has dementia may only lead to frustration and anger. Dementia takes away the full ability to think logically but they are still a person and arguing is never fun.

2) Don't Stop! Just because an action may be against the norm is it really an issue? Think about whether it is a real problem. If it is not harmful and makes them happy, let them carry on. Try joining them and discovering a new part of their persona.

3) Don't Boss! Becoming a carer does not give anyone authority over another person. Don't try to control their actions to the point where they lose their free will. They are still a person.

4) Don't Dismiss! There is a popular movement that I believe originated on Twitter "Nothing about me, without me". If a decision needs to be made involving them, they should be involved. Likewise for conversations, if it can be held around them they should be encouraged to take part. They are still a person.

5) Enter their world. Often a person with dementia will be creating and living in a world separate to our reality. This is usually harmless and it can really benefit them to have

this world acknowledged. They are still a person.

6) Give options and celebrate the achievements made, no matter how small a task may be for us, for a person with dementia it can be infinitely more difficult. Having successes acknowledged helps build confidence. Ask for and value their opinion. They are still a person.

7) Live with Open Eyes. Be able to spot, intercept and avert causes of agitation and stress. These can be caused by a multitude of things including but not limited to: Too much noise, activity, clutter, unfamiliar people and places, sudden movements, feeling of loss or insecurity. Being asked several questions at once, responding to arguments amongst others, responding to impatience, stress, irritability, being scolded/confronted/contradicted, being surprised, discovering inability to complete tasks, receiving unclear instructions, changing schedules, short attention span, and task not broken down. They are still a person, and being overwhelmed is stressful.

8) Give them time to be alone. No one wants to feel imprisoned and both a carer and caree need breathing space. They are still a person and are entitled to having space to think (if safe).

9) Cherish the person. Don't just focus on the dementia, which is merely an aspect of the person. Treat them in a way we would wish to be treated. They are still a person.

10) Remember the three things we all deserve: Respect, Dignity, and Freedom. We are all people.

Chapter 7:

July 2013:

"A good day. No scrap that. A pigging wonderful day. Started off being awakened by a call from my Admiral Nurse. She wanted to know if I'd like to meet up today. Well in about an hour. Yes I did. So scrambled out of bed and just about made it on time. I know I mention this a lot but I really do love my Admiral Nurse. She gives me the nudges and pushes, along with a professional opinion and a cosy chat. I honestly think we need more of her around!

Anyway she was pleased to hear about Nan's involvement in recent activities and about how well work is going. She gave me a few tips about how to avoid purse hunting in the middle of the night (replica purses, make sure she has purse as putting her to bed) and encouraged me to look into advanced education because caring is something I'm good at and enjoy.

So I came home feeling pumped and finally decided to get round to the life book. I invited Nan upstairs to help me do the ironing and thought she could look at photos while I got on, but I was far too easily distracted and so we spent 3 hours sitting chatting about the photos, the situations and me furiously scribbling every word Nan said!

So we now have the photos, accompanied by some statements (which will be typed up and will follow in the next blog).

I then showed Nan how to send a tweet and she loved it so much she had another go unsupervised.

Such a proud carer and granddaughter today, and we both feel happier.

And that big black cloud of doom I felt approaching? He's buggered off to where he belongs. In that pit I dug a few months ago and have recently filled in and covered up in the hopes of not falling down again.

So far Nan and I have enjoyed knitting together. Nan has been struggling with pain in her wrists though, as she is like me and refuses to stop. We each have our own knitting needles and now I'm a bit more competent Nan likes to watch me.

We watched a video the other day on how to knit a hat. I thought this would be ideal for my dad's birthday so we got started. Easy enough knit knit, knit knit. Then we had to reduce. Nan couldn't remember how and the video wasn't easy to understand so we just made it up.

In hindsight, that's probably where I went wrong. Nan decided not to reduce and just carried on knitting. I however made a royal blunder and now my hat has ended up looking like a teeny witch's hat."

Days like this could keep me going for weeks. The days where we spend the whole time laughing and joking, where Nanny Jean rips me to shreds with her wit. This particular days bliss carried on for several after because every time one of us passed by the giant Mickey Mouse in the corner we would crack up again. Mickey Mouse had been chosen as the lucky recipient of the witch's hat and he still sits as a gentle reminder of the good times we have had. And a reminder that Nan isn't just about the dementia, despite the odds she taught me, a stubborn, impatient, awkward fool, how to knit. And that really is quite the achievement, for both of us.

Feeling Worthwhile/Something to live for:

It is so important for us humans to feel like we have a purpose, and for those with dementia even more so. I would hate to think that Nan feels like she is losing a reason for living because she does not feel worthwhile. During my time as a carer, and through conversations with other carers and experts, I have found 3 things that can encourage feelings of fulfilment and purpose and would like to share them.

The first is pets. Nan has her cat, and me my rabbit. When I am having a horrible day where I could just hide in bed all day and not face life I think of my poor (fat) bunny possibly starving away because I haven't fed him since last night. The cuddles he gives and the way he looks at me (yes he talks too!) certainly make me feel more positive about the day. He also gives great man advice, being a man himself. I find Nan has the same feelings about the cat, he is someone to talk to when I am not around, and she takes more care ensuring he is fed than she does herself. He not only gives her companionship, but a reason to get up out of the chair and walk around, using instinct to find out what he wants. He seems to sense that nan needs more love than I do, he will bypass me most days to talk to nan, and glare at me when I come in, (possibly because I tried to change his name, nan just calls him boy now as she forgot his name when she was in hospital). I think having a pet can give some stability and routine, to an otherwise dull and possibly lonely life.

There is currently a scheme involving "dementia dogs" which I have been reading about, and feel there are many benefits to. If a caree does not have their own pet it may be worthwhile doing some research into the dogs. This way in the event of them needing to stay in hospital they are still able to take photos of the pet to interact with and this could keep them stimulated, as well as giving them more incentive to go home (nan was determined to get out of hospital to come home and feed "boy"). I am aware however that this could cause distress and worry, so it is important to be sensitive to a caree's thoughts and wishes.

The second thing that I've heard can help people living with dementia is dolls. There has of course been some controversy about whether it is right to encourage carees to re-enact a childlike state by "playing" with toys. But I see it as more than that. And luckily others do too. It becomes more than playing, the doll becomes real (but is slightly more robust and so much better than a real baby for those in the later stages of dementia). They not only provide comfort but also that sense of purpose and the ability to feel worthwhile that we all crave. Dolls can prompt maternal instincts and there are many articles about the successes of using them in care homes.

The third thing I found to help us all live a life where we feel worthwhile was brought to my attention through a chat on social network. Compliments. For all of us receiving a compliment can brighten up our day, and remembering compliments is a great way to prevent getting down. I remember when I was having a rough time and had low self-esteem it was recommended that I write down compliments I had been given and tell them to myself in the mirror every-time I hit a wall. If other people think these great things about me I should too.

And this works the other way round as well. To be forgetting how to undertake what used to be simple tasks, and parts of what makes a person themselves, must be devastating. And this can occur for a person living with dementia when clarity hits and they realise that there is something "wrong" with them. The best way to help here is to buoy them up with compliments on the things they can do, and have achieved (like Nan with her knitting). Another nice idea is to tell them often how enjoyable it is being with them, how well a task they've done is, how nice they look today, just how bloody brilliant they are.

It is important to remember that this is not just applicable to the caree. As demonstrated from the following passage from my blog:

"And remember you are too, even if no one else tells you, I will. I think you are all fantastic, however big or small your part is in caring for someone, you are making a difference. And it is appreciated.

"There are no small parts, only small actors"- I'm going to twist the meaning to fit in here, but no part of caring is small, from 24h care to long distance to visiting relatives once a week/month. You can make yourself small by putting down the things you do. So go on, smile, lift your chin up and feel worthwhile. I sure think you are."

Chapter 8:

August 2013:

> ""Hello my name is John and I'm calling from
> National Accident Helpline"
> .... "Hello my name is David and I'm calling
> from National Accident Helpline"

After several of these calls the last couple of days (seven between today and yesterday) I am unashamed to admit I truly lost it down the phone to John/Dave (pretty sure it was the same guy anyway).

The first time he called I explained very politely we had not had any accidents and would like our number to be removed from the system. We ended up having a dispute, I mentioned I was a carer for the home owner and so he refused to speak to me, insisting he needed to speak to the home owner. I calmly explained she had dementia and so any deals to be done were to be done through me. And that as neither of us has had an accident could he not call again. We went through the same conversation FOUR TIMES! Before I hung up, frustrated that still, no one seems to accept a carer's point in life.

Every time he has called since I have told him to remove our number before giving him a chance to speak and then hung up. What annoys me is how they keep calling, I have a feeling they are hoping to catch Nan when I am not there so they can scam her. I dread to think what Nan would agree to if she answered, she can barely understand a London accent, let alone an Indian one.

But the seventh call tonight was too much. I shouted, I swore and I threatened to shred his telephone line if he calls again. Have reported National Accident Helpline as a Spam company, but I doubt this will achieve anything as even being on the "list of unspammable numbers" hasn't helped. I appreciate everyone needs a job, but if some-one says no, they tend to mean no.

I just thought I'd give you all an update on Nan. She's doing well, as am I. It's just this week she seems to have realised there's something "wrong" with her. I don't like using the word wrong, it makes it seem as though I am disagreeing with the way Dementia Nan does things, and it makes her abnormal somehow. And that's not what I mean. But Nan does seem to have realised that it's not me moving things, or things walking off etc. but that these things are happening on her part (or Dementia Nan's part).

And I'm not sure how that makes me feel. Does that mean she is developing more into the later stages of dementia now she is past the denial stage? Is it good that she now realises she is not as capable as she was when she was just Nanny Jean? I feel guilty of course, that if I'd done something different she could have remained in ignorant bliss a little while longer. I worry that now she thinks there's something "wrong" she'll stop trying. I want to keep her as active and stimulated as long as possible, but I have a fine line of trying not to let her think she's invincible. Partly I'm being selfish, I won't let Nan go without a fight, as I feel I've put so much hard work into keeping the dementia from affecting her too much. So seeing the sudden dips spurs me on. But mostly I want to protect her, from herself, or dementia self.

So I've upped my game. Took her down the village this morning and encouraged her to choose something, and pay for it herself. She bought herself some cookies, and refused to let me carry them to the car. Put them lovingly in her biscuit box and has not stopped snacking all day. This afternoon I encouraged Nan to help with the ironing, which she did with a smile on her face (more than I can manage when I'm ironing!).

Then we attempted social media again, this time on the laptop to see if she found it easier. I'm going to try and play around with the screen size so she can see what she is typing easier. But once I explained it was more like a typewriter she was whizzing away, and I didn't have to prompt sentences. It was great to see her thinking out a one way conversation and something I really would like to pursue with her. Considering an old laptop for her for Christmas. But we'll see how we go.

I still get cross when I think of all the nuisance calls, and despite changing our number and re-adding ourselves to the mythical list of un spammable numbers we still get at least one phone call a day from various companies checking our windows, conservatory, computer and insurance needs. I have read up on some great ways to prank them though, (without making their lives hell, I am still trying to keep in mind that we all need to make a living).

Nanny Jean has dipped a few times since I wrote this post. She seems completely unaware of many things, and has forgotten some of herself such as foods she enjoys and who her relatives are. When asked questions she turns them back so she doesn't have to answer and gives one or two standard responses to literally anything I say. It is hard to get her full attention and her physical responses have been weakened. She no longer has the strength or co-ordination to walk unaided (particularly after sun down) and has a lot more Dementia Nan moments where she becomes unpleasant to be around (in the sense of being venomous and spiteful, we are lucky that she is not physically abusive).

I have included at the end of the book Nanny Jean's latest attempt at typing, it was not only the writing she struggled with but also the thinking of what to type. Asking Nanny Jean to complete a task where there is more than one action will result in nothing getting done and an increasingly stressed Nan. She is also starting to see people who are invisible to the rest of us, and can be heard telling them how much the rest of the family distrusts them when she has the energy to wander around the house.

So we've adapted our approaches. Everything is broken down as much as it can be, including food which she now struggles to chew and swallow. Questions are kept basic. Security cameras have been installed that can alert us via our phones if something is wrong. The carers come in more regularly and do a few more tasks, like putting toothpaste on the toothbrush as Nan can't hold the brush and work the tube at the same time. But above all we don't act like anything is different, this is our new normal.

And Nanny Jean is happy chatting nonsense to the cat for hours. She seems happy to let me waffle with her, as long as we maintain eye contact and she gets a chance to nod or drop in a generic sentence. Most importantly Nanny Jean is still here, living with dementia, not suffering.

Communication/Can I Be Heard?

Learning Something New:

"The first few times we saw the Talent advert I could see Nan searching her head for the right words, and then the other day "would you believe I used to do that". "What nan?" "Acrobatics". Wow. I was shocked, Nan has often mentioned to me her love of dancing but I had never heard this story. I am aware that sometimes people with dementia often believe that the things they have seen have happened to them, so I took the new story with a pinch of salt. But it was fascinating to see Nan chatting with enthusiasm about this old hobby.

This conversation lead us on to the dancing she used to do, at the London Palladium would you believe! But due to the War starting she had to stop as she was evacuated. And then I heard all about her two failed evacuations and the return to her mum in the city. Nan spent most of the evening chatting to me about her past, with me listening, which was nice as I often feel I do most of the talking.

The following day I thought it would be nice for Nan to see some of her old things, jewelry and postcards etc. Unfortunately Nan's memory was not on top form so the stories I had been hoping for did not come, but she smiled fondly at old relics of her past, and gave me a few hints of a time gone by."

This old post brings me to the point of this part of the chapter. One of the many lessons I learned from Jennie the Admiral Nurse was not to force a person living with dementia to live in the present.

Allow them to live and believe in the things they believe are real, as long as they are not a risk to themselves or others.

It is possible to learn a lot by doing this. Nanny Jean has not developed that far into her dementia, she is still vaguely aware of the present day (at least I think she is, she just doesn't know what/when present day is) but I believe that at some point she will regress – she already thinks she is twenty years younger, which I suppose would make this the 90's. And I think I'm prepared for that, to allow her to live in the past may teach me things I was never aware of. We all need to be aware of how much we can truly learn from our elders, as often they are ignored or listened to but not truly heard. I never knew my nan did acrobatics, or that my grandma lived on a farm in Folkstone (pretty much the frontline of raids) during the war, so had supplies of milk etc. while a family friend struggled through the rationing up in Yorkshire (far from the raids).

When working with or talking to children, we try to keep them in their childhood world, with their imaginary friends for as long as it keeps them happy. If we wouldn't destroy that world, or tell that child that their best friend isn't real why would we do it for someone living with dementia?

The more I interacted with Nanny Jean, the more I listened and asked the right questions, the more I learned. Our frankest discussion, which needed to be had, came after a rather spectacular meltdown on my part over some sandwiches:

Unfortunately I have been finding it hard to not snap lately, and the straw that broke the camel's back was sandwiches. I know in hindsight it is pathetic of me to get so cross over the sandwiches but at the time they represented so much more than plain old cheese sandwiches.

We have been asking the carers to prepare some sandwiches so that Nan has something to eat to tide her over until the evening carers come, and in case I go out. However after a few days it became apparent that Nan was hiding the sandwiches in the bin" (Yes I meant hiding, they would be wrapped in kitchen towel, newspaper and then placed under various other objects), *"or picking the cheese out and throwing the bread away. After a week of observing the sandwiches not being eaten I asked Nan why she wasn't finishing them (forgetting the cardinal rule from the Admiral Nurse – don't question behaviours). She got rather snappy about it, saying she has been eating them.*

And I'm ashamed to say this flipped my switch, and all the concerns I've been keeping to myself, and the worries I have about her came flooding out. About how I'm concerned if she doesn't eat she'll get ill, end up in hospital and not be allowed home, if the social think I'm not taking good enough care of her they'll put her in a home, she might fall if there is no one here to look after her, and as she has previous for leaving the grill/hob on I'm scared she'll set the house on fire. Needless to say my rant did not go down well, and it took me a good half hour of apologising to get Nan to look at me again, let alone talk to me. I can't say I blame her, she's spent 80 years being a perfectly capable person and to be told someone thinks you are no longer able of doing some of the most simple tasks must be awful.

Nan also told me she feels like a prisoner sometimes, and that hurt me because I'm trying to help her have as much of a normal life as possible, whilst trying to protect her, I don't want her to feel trapped. So then we sat down and had a big heart to heart, all the things she wants and needs and how we can achieve them as well as keeping her safe. She was much more honest with me than she was with the social, which is to be expected I guess but was still nice to hear. After a couple of hours we decided to drop the weekday carers and I will take over their duties. And at the weekends I will leave her with the carers to go out. We discussed activities that Nan wants to do, and a few things I can do to help her feel more independent."

There's a reason the Admiral Nurse gave me golden rules for caring for a person with dementia, the above goes to show just how resentful I was becoming by not letting go of the smaller things, by not listening to Nanny Jean. If I had asked her from the start what she wanted instead of mollycoddling her we could have avoided a lot of drama. But I was so determined to not fail, or admit that I was struggling that I took it all upon myself, and tended to forget so many of the rules that could have helped keep us both sane.

Chapter 9:

September 2013:

"Songs really seem to resonate with me, which is why so many of my posts include song lyrics and titles. I find it easier to sum up my feelings with a song, or by writing it down. The words can't come out of my mouth right and I end up sounding rude or ungrateful.

Feeling much more positive today after my breakdown Tuesday. It's so easy to lose the way with caring, especially with dementia. Even more so if we forget why we're here. It took a few people to kick me up the arse. Virtual friends and real life ones, both as important as each other for me. To keep me on the path as far away from a meltdown as possible. I'm here to help not only Nan but myself, and yes some days it sucks. And yes there are things on hold. But I shouldn't and won't let them get away without me.

Dementia Nan makes things seem so stormy for me and I can't even begin to imagine how it must be in Nan's head. We assume those with dementia just forget everything, and so don't realise the effects. But it's not like that at all. They don't forget everything. First of all, it's been proven that muscle remembers actions (hence Nan being able to knit) plus she remembers events from days long gone and from recent years. Sometimes she even remembers that she has asked a question many repeatedly, that she used to be able to do this and now she can't. Worst of all she remembers who she was, and is struggling to accept that she is not completely that person anymore. I try to help in what little ways I can by encouraging her to be that person, but there are physical limitations as well as the wearing effects of the dementia. And so she is trying to come to terms with saying goodbye to parts of herself.

And I suppose I am too, goodbye to parts of her and to parts of me (not all of which I am sorry to lose- that stone in weight was a welcome goodbye, the selfishness and superficiality of so many things I used to enjoy are two traits I am also glad to lose). But to re iterate the point from the Brenner's – This is also a time to say hello. And I think this will work better once Nan has accepted her "loss". We can find new things to enjoy, and new ways of doing things. We can both become new people together on this journey and enjoy it all the more because we are doing it together."

The Brenner's wrote a fantastic book that helped me through accepting Nan's dementia. Their main point, which is one I have become passionate about is that dementia isn't all about saying a long goodbye to someone. There is a great opportunity for reinvention, not only for the caree but also for people like me, I could be who I wanted to be, who Nan wanted me to be, and I learned a lot about myself and my future goals in the process.

Listen With Your Heart - non-verbal communication:

Following on from the last chapter regarding verbal communication I think I should also cover the importance of non-verbal communication. The importance of being able to anticipate the emotional highs and lows of a loved one with dementia. I don't expect anybody to become mind readers. But there are ways of noticing how a person is feeling without the need for them to verbalize. Verbal messages become more and more difficult for someone with dementia so it can be hard to adapt to look for nonverbal signals if they have not already been associated while the person is vocal. Here are some examples I look for with Nan;

* Arms crossed – This tends to mean that Nanny Jean is cold. Depending on the time of year this could be a trigger for the heating to go on or fetching a cup of tea and a blanket (because who can afford to have the heating on in July)?!

* Stroking or patting her hair – Nan does not agree with what is being said. Or has lost interest. The best thing to do here is to change the subject of conversation, or offer chocolate.

* Peering at the clock – This one seems self-explanatory. Nanny Jean wants to know the time. As I have mentioned previously people who are living with dementia can find it to be a struggle to understand what the clock means. We have tried a digital clock with a large face but Nanny Jean wanted that one in

her bedroom. So we are stuck with the miniature grandfather clock (the one with the tiny face that even I struggle to read). But Nanny Jean is attached to it so I'm loathe to change it. If I see Nan looking at the clock I tell her the time, and then the scheduled programming for the hour (Memorising the television book really did come in handy!)

* Dusting – If Nan starts cleaning I know she is getting agitated. She may not know or understand why that is, but I think that most of the time it is down to frustration at not knowing what to do with herself. This is when I get out her life book to read and talk about, or find a game to play. Or join her with housework if it needs doing (I will try and find a million other things to do first though).

* Slamming drawers – If I hear more than two drawers being shut I know that Nanny Jean has lost something. This is where I use my lightning quick reflexes and intercept as quickly as possible. If Nan looks in more than a couple of places she tends to forget what she is looking for and then becomes very upset.

* Cupping her face – I had to ask Nan about this one as it looks like a very uncomfortable position to sit in for long periods of time, and I assumed she had tooth ache. But apparently this is a comfort to her, and means she is relaxed.

* Nanny death stare – This is infamous throughout our family and something we often

joke about. If anybody receives this look a horrific atrocity has been committed and must be rectified immediately. This is when I scuttle out to get fish and chips.

* Invading personal space – Nan and I are not overly touchy people, so I know that if she comes within two feet of me she wants a cuddle, or has picked up on my deeper emotions and thinks I need one. Honestly her intuition is not to be messed with.

* Refusing food – When Nanny Jean tells me she is not hungry it means she is in pain, but is unwilling to admit she is bothered by it. This is frustrating for me as I know she needs food to keep up her strength. As Nan once worked in a hospital she is aware that most medications need food to work properly. This is the way we compromise, painkillers in exchange for food.

I have also discovered that occasionally I can tell whether Nanny Jean is herself or whether she is under the cloud of Dementia Nan (I found the same thing with a couple of clients). She almost looks like a different person and that has made it easier to avoid confrontation:

"So after a bit of a dip Nan and I are much more positive today. I came home yesterday and she had been using the stove, something I would prefer was not done when I'm not here due to the near misses in the past (dishcloth soup anyone)? *Kept my emotions under control and just left her eating her dinner. I'm not sure how but I could tell it was*

Dementia Nan sitting in the chair not Nanny Jean. So I went and stewed upstairs until I was certain Nan was back."

These are not the only methods of nonverbal communication that I use to interpret Nanny Jean, there are of course the obvious ones such as head movements and eye rolls, as well as others such as hand tapping, tutting and pacing but if I listed everything I would have a whole other book. Every person is unique so the meanings that are attached to Nanny Jean may not necessarily apply to somebody else. It is important to get to know a person's habits in order to prevent harmful or damaging situations, and to make communication and listening easier in the case of a deterioration of verbal skills.

Chapter 10

October 2013

"So I've actually missed writing but a few outside factors have interfered with me updating as regularly as I would like. Firstly Dementia Nan is making more frequent appearances, so Nanny Jean and I are having to make adjustments. Secondly I've been living my life. I spent a whole day out with a friend, popped home to make dinner and then went back out to the cinema for the night. Then I did the memory walk, and thanks to everyone who donated, we raised £220. Which has spurred me on to do more to raise awareness and funds for dementia, Alzheimer's and carers' charities and organisations. Let me know if you can think of any funny, original ideas for my next challenge. Then of course I had my well needed trip to Disneyland!

So the dementia. Hasn't been a barrel of laughs but there have been highlights, like covering each other's faces in chocolate mousse. Just because. Of course there are the down sides, Nan is struggling to remember the names of anyone in the family that she doesn't talk to everyday, and you can see it pains her to admit she's struggling. And as winter is nearly upon us we have started back up with the "looks like rain" comments, and the daily fights about the heating. However I am coping much better than last year and am learning to let the frustrations slide right off.

I think it helps that I am finding more balance, more time for myself and not feeling so guilty about work or socialising. The world hasn't ended yet! Nan is finding day to day life harder, I've noticed her struggling more with where things are, how to start a task and generally requiring a bit more prompting. But we're working round it.

Archery helped, and I'm entering a competition in a couple of weeks. Seriously doubt I'll be any good as I hadn't shot for three months but it'll be nice to get back on track."

*   *   *

"Who is Neil?"

"This is a question I have been asking myself over and over tonight. I got in from work and Nan had left me a note to say Neil had called round. Wonderful. But I'm not sure I know a Neil! Of course she couldn't remember what he looked like, or what he had knocked for. But when I checked she had some money missing. And so of course she was getting worked up, despite me trying to keep it all behind her back.

It may of course be completely innocent. Neil may be completely harmless, but when you care for someone and these things happen it really does put you off of ever leaving the house.

That would be ridiculous however. Tempted as I am to lock Nan in and wrap her in bubble wrap it won't do either of us any good limiting our freedoms. I'd like to think she learns from her mistakes, but now she can't remember anything happening today at all.

Which I'm grateful for, I'd rather she felt calm and peaceful (someone should). But I wish there was a way to stop her letting any old random in (this happened yesterday when she let a fella in, just because he knew my name. Fortunately it was harmless but did lead to me talking to someone I should probably have kept in the past)."

Looking back I can see how much progress I had made as a carer in just the ten months I was blogging. When I first started I had no idea what I was doing, Nan was new to being cared for and we didn't communicate enough to understand each other's' needs.

Back in January I thought it was best for Nan that I do everything for her and wrap her up to keep her from experiencing the possibility of any harm. Nan still thought she could be independent and saw me coming in as a threat to her freedom. And that is what I was doing. It took me too long to realise that Nan did need to do things for herself, that she was perfectly capable of surviving a day without me smothering her.

Around October I stopped writing as often as I had been, looking back I suppose that it was a sign that we were both coping better. I no longer needed to rant as much, and I was starting to take on board the lessons I had learned.

And I was starting to let go, giving Nan the opportunity to experiment with what she felt capable of doing. And I really believe that this started to happen after our conversation from the previous chapter, it shouldn't have happened in the way it did, but it did need to happen. Life became much easier for both of us after a frank discussion about any changes that needed to be made.

Unfortunately during my time caring for Nanny Jean, mostly during the year of my blog, I forgot to take care of myself. And this lead to situations that were uncomfortable for both of us, and I'm fairly certain I made life much more difficult than Nan needed it to be.

I'm a Bitch/Why you should care for yourself

The following are examples of the too many situations where I exploded and I wanted to share them, as hard as it is to relive them. Because every carer I have spoken to goes through these moments, it's a combination of stress, guilt, fatigue and neglecting ourselves. They happen, and it is important to accept why they are happening and how to prevent them, rather than concealing them due to being ashamed.

"Well tonight has been what can only be described as hellish. I could have quite happily packed my bags and roamed the streets. It all started because Nan had gone upstairs. I hate this when I go out" (the stairs were exceptionally steep with a concrete floor at the bottom, basically a cracked skull waiting to happen-especially for someone like me who is prone to thinking the worst) *"so it's one of our three golden rules. I was feeling on edge and so didn't handle it as well as I should have. I know it's my fault and I let rip. Dementia Nan was attacking me with all the 'you make me feel like a prisoner' 'I don't need you here, what do you I couldn't?'*

There are things I think sometimes in my darkest moments. Things I don't tell anybody. Things I always hoped Nan never knew. But I flipped. And told Dementia Nan that I wasn't sure why I had put my life on hold for her, nobody else had or would. That if it wasn't for me she'd be in a care home by now. And that sometimes I think she'd be better off there as she's so miserable with me. That it wasn't choice that sent me to her and I didn't have to keep doing it. And that's when Nan can back. And burst into tears.

And because I'm so awful that just made me feel crosser. So I had to leave the room. I was sick of constantly worrying about Dementia Nan and her feelings. I wanted to wallow in mine. So I ended up stewing in my twisted, guilty messed up head and feeling worse.

I apologised and my mum got involved to act as a peace keeper. Things still feel on edge but maybe it's me. I don't want people to think I'm a good carer who copes so well because I don't think I am. Deep down I fear I'm becoming resentful, not only of Nan but of all those people I know who are getting to do what they want to do, living the lives they want.

I feel conflicted. I want to stick by Nan. And I know this is just a blip. But how many more blips do I stick with before I leave the table?"

I had so many moments where I doubted myself, whether I really was doing what was right for Nan, or if I was in fact making things harder for her. Looking back I know most of the time I was helping, that I did have a positive impact, but if I was going to do it again I would make more of a conscious decision to look after myself. This way I could prevent situations like this from happening again.

"Still feeling guilty today about an outburst yesterday. I completely snapped. Got in from work, feeling tired. Did my usual checks through the house and couldn't find Nan's purse. Getting quite worked up about it, we used to have one hiding place and now

it seems there is about 50. And all the time I was searching Nan was hovering, and questioning. "What are you doing?" "Why do you want my purse?" "What are you looking for?" Finally found the purse and as I was checking through it Nan was hovering right over me. "What are you doing, what are you doing? What are you doing? Why have you got my purse? What are you doing with my money? Why are you taking my money?" And I flipped. I told her to leave me alone, I had just got in from work, I was tired and I shouldn't have to get in from work to hunt for things that should be kept in the same place. And as I was trying to help her, I would appreciate not being accused of stealing and could she please just go and sit down and leave me alone for five minutes.

Ordinarily I would have coped very well with this situation, just auto piloting the same sentence of reassurance. But yesterday I had had enough. I wanted some me time, true genuine me time.

I did apologise. And of course Nan couldn't remember once dinner was made. But I still feel foul. Like a truly horrible person. It's been a while since I flipped at Nan, and I thought I was able to get out of those situations and handle them better.

I understand though that it's normal, and I guess, OK to have days where you can't handle any more interrogations, invasions of personal space, or whatever it is that triggers you. It just makes me feel guilty that I can't be this perfect superman figure, who has it all worked out.

I guess we all have our cracks, just some people keep them well hidden. And others crack on the surface, for everyone to see. And why should I hide my cracks? They are a part of my relationship with Nan, as much as the dementia is."

The great (I use this word very loosely) thing about dementia is that when Dementia Nan and I have an argument, Nanny Jean doesn't remember it happening. (That's not to say that arguing with her is acceptable, or justified). So we can wake up the next day as if nothing has happened, well from her perspective anyway. I end up feeling slightly bitter, but of course I conceal it and don't act on it because that would confuse and upset Nanny Jean. So as ever, carry on regardless, the theme of living with dementia, or supporting a caree who is living with it. Carry on as if there is nothing out of the ordinary. And don't sweat too much about cracking occasionally, dementia is a very high intensity roommate.

Chapter 11:

November 2013

"Hello all, apologies once again for another long break. I fell ill with a cold/man flu/the Black Death and haven't felt much up to anything. Which has been convenient as Nan also fell poorly this week. Yet another infection which has left her more confused, tired, cold and generally miserable. Suffice to say the atmosphere hasn't been great in the house. So I asked mum to take Nan out for a drive to give us both a break from each other.

I'm still not sleeping right, nothing worrying me or stressing me out. But the moon, it's just so damn bright! I'm almost missing the sleepy town, even the bright lights of London. The eerie glow of a streetlight is much easier to sleep to than the shiny shininess of the moon. And of course I have to sit up and look at it, and all the stars. There's so many here, and then I play games like "plane/star/superman" "falling star/u.f.o" which have kept me wide awake until at least 3am. Meanwhile Nan is absolutely soundo from ten til nine every night, leading to me feeling resentful that she's sleeping so well! Of course though I'm glad she is, she clearly needs it.

Anyway back to today, Nan went off with mum and I decided to make the most of my morning alone. I did want to dance around naked, but I'm unsure the bloke fitting the kitchen would have been too impressed. So I knitted. And watched a DVD, and watched Doctor Who again. And listened to McFly. And sat and twiddled my thumbs. Is this how people feel when their kids go off to school? Is that why they always end up with another baby on the way? What on earth am I supposed to do? Couldn't relax as felt so restless! But did enjoy not having to answer incessant questions.

Mum then came to pick me up and we went out for lunch. It was gorgeous and we were all getting along splendidly, until halfway through pudding when Nan just stopped eating. Mum asked if she was ok and Nan suddenly went very green. And pulled *that* sick face. That was my cue to push my chair away from the table and run. And mum got up very suddenly, both of us leaving Nan to heave in her chair. Mum and I had a brief argument (I say brief it felt like it went on for hours, but can't have been more than a minute) of who would take nan outside and who would pay the bill, as when it comes to vomit we are both absolute wusses. I lost and patted Nan on the back as I hurried her outside, my usually caring nature completely collapsing and leaving me feeling paranoid that Nan was going to vomit on me. Found a chair outside and sat Nan down, and as politely as I could took a few steps away. Did the only thing I can do when I feel awkward and made jokes, Nan laughed but looked so fragile.

When we got home Nan got straight into bed and fell asleep, so I did some research into the meds the doctor prescribed for her infection. Was there anything she shouldn't have eaten? Side effects? Was I a bad person for not reading the leaflet before giving them to Nan? I felt cross (and told mum so) that mum pushed vomit duty onto me, and then felt cross at myself for being horrible. Nan was poorly and I was thinking about myself. I discovered the meds should not be given to someone with kidney problems, which is the reason they were prescribed. So the doctor will be called in the morning to find out what is going on. In the meantime I think we'll avoid the meds.

Nan woke up after a 4 and a half hour sleep saying she felt a bit better but still nauseous, so we chilled on the sofa and had a giggle."

This makes me chuckle every time I read it, I can just see mum's face as she realises what's happening, knowing that is the exact same expression that was on my face. I know for a fact that if this were to happen again it would be the exact same fight, and I'd lose again and be on vomit duty. Poor Nan, I'd do a lot for her. I conquered my hatred of feet to cut her toenails and help her put her tights on. I overcame my issues about seeing her naked and helped her to wash. I've wiped her bottom. I've cleaned poop (both cat and human) off the floor. I've sterilised and plastered open wounds. I worked with babies and dealt with some unnatural nappy disasters. But if Nan ever vomits near me I think she'll be on her own with me outside the door making soothing noises while holding my nose and trying to cover my ears.

Depression/living in darkness

"Help, I need somebody. Help, not just anybody. Help, you know I need someone. When I was younger so much younger than today. I never needed anybody's help in anyway. But now those days are gone, I'm not so self-assured. And now I find, I've changed my mind, I've opened up the doors. Help me if you can I'm feeling down, and I do appreciate you being round. Help me get my feet back on the ground. Won't you please, please help me? And now my life has changed in oh so many ways, my independence seems to have vanished in the haze. But every now and then I feel so insecure, I know that I just need you like, I've never done before..." – lyrics belong to the Beatles, but I was listening to the Mcfly version.

"It's ok to sometimes feel like you want to scream. Or run away. I know this because I have been feeling this way. Many times lately I could have happily got in my car and driven into the horizon. Nothing in particular has triggered it, but I feel like I'm stuck in a pit, spinning round and round trying to find an exit. But I can't see the exit because I'm spinning so fast. It's a normal reaction to an abnormal situation; no money, no job and the pressure of caring are abnormal situations, and thrown all together are something else entirely. I suppose recently I have been worrying about when the worst happens. What happens when Nan dies? I feel like I'll lose all focus and purpose in life, she is currently everything I have. Everything I do I am thinking about Nan and the impact for her, and when that is taken away I'm worried of how I'll cope.

I saw my Admiral Nurse this week and mentioned how I'd been feeling, and she reassured me so well I nearly broke down in the middle of the coffee shop. She helped me realise that there are things I can do to help myself. Rule Number 1 as a carer: Remember to care for yourself. For those of you currently in a pit with me, I want you all to know there is an exit to the pit, just climb out. It'll be hard work but it's possible, you just have to stop spinning long enough to see it.

To avoid depression and stress whilst caring, the Admiral Nurse told me there are three things you need in your life. Sleep, 3 healthy meals a day, and exercise. All of which I have been ignoring lately. For a good nights sleep, make sure you have a bedtime routine. And if you can't sleep don't worry about it, it's nothing you weren't missing in the first place. And the anxiety of not sleeping will be keeping the adrenaline pumping, keeping you awake. Lavender oil and warm milk can really help. Make sure you are eating well enough to keep your body going, healthy body healthy mind and all that! And exercise, it doesn't have to be much, a five minute walk can do wonders, or even just exercising in the garden.

The Admiral Nurse also gave me some homework this week. I have to make a list of all the amazing things I have achieved to look at when I feel low. I was a little sceptical, currently I feel like everything I do fails, or I could have done better (damn the pit). But she made me think. Every carer should do this list. Because we are amazing. There are alternatives but we chose to do this for our loved ones. Which makes us amazing. My admiral nurse told me so. We are constantly learning and by sharing our experiences we are doing something else amazing. Educating and supporting others.

So remember, YOU ARE AMAZING!!! I have so much love for all of you, carers or not, if you're reading this you're supporting not only me, but all my other readers too. So once again I thank you for reading and sharing.

PS It is OK to ask for help!!!

UPDATE: What a difference a day makes (or a night in my case, one good night's sleep). After seeing the Admiral Nurse I kicked myself up the bottom, bought some lavender, after a recommendation from a Twitter follower I bought some Chamomile Tea and I went out to see a friend. I was exhausted when I got back (probably due to not really having been out much lately) but I felt amazing. So I would like to thank her for uplifting me and putting the spring back in my step. And then I slept, all night. Did not wake once. I know that these solutions will not work for everybody, and I know that getting out is not always feasible. But I really would suggest it to anyone feeling low, especially carers who do not get much time alone. I have been feeling not great, but OK for the last couple of days, and definitely feel more capable of tackling a few more days!"

As it turns out I was only concentrating on short term recovery, and as such would feel good for a couple of days before falling back down into my pit. It isn't quite as simple as "just climbing out" but it is important to recognise that these issues are just my mind playing tricks on me. I had to change my thought processes, which takes a while and a lot of conscious effort. But I find that when I tell myself that these thoughts are not my own and are not welcome I can distance myself from them long enough to make some progress in climbing up.

Climbing up for me is made much easier once I start making myself do something. For example going for a walk, just a short twenty minute blast of fresh air can help clear my thoughts and gets my blood pumping long enough to remind me that I'm alive. I always found the problem with the depression though was the getting started and getting outside in the first place, so I broke everything down. I will just get dressed and see how I feel. I will open the door to check the weather. I will walk to the end of the drive. I will walk to the next street lamp. By breaking it down into shorter tasks I convinced myself to make progress. It will not be the same for everybody though, and I would urge anyone with similar issues to seek help from a doctor.

*   *   *

"This is something I have fretted about discussing, seeing as how I haven't kept my blog particularly anonymous for myself. But if I can't be honest, than why should anyone else? The whole idea of this blog was to get people to open up, so that dementia could become less of a taboo. It has been great to see this in effect, with all the supportive messages I have received, as well as the messages of gratitude from those I have helped. This in turn has prompted me to speak out about other issues. Namely, the other "big D" in my life. "Depression".

When I was younger it was something I admit I struggled with, but I guess in recent years I put it down to teenage mood swings (as did the people around me) because I had started coping so well. Recently though I could feel the old emotions creeping back (as I mentioned in a previous post-feeling like

I'm in a dark pit, spinning and spinning with no way to escape). To elaborate, I feel like a failure. Nothing I can do seems to help Nan, and she still feels like a prisoner. I can't seem to get a job, despite having a degree so I must be pretty useless on that front. My thoughts become more and more negative, to the point where I don't want to see my friends (sorry guys), it's just too much effort to smile and laugh. I don't want to leave the house because I feel like a failure on the outside (I need to lose weight, my skin is awful, my hair is greasy etc. etc.) as well as emotionally.

Thankfully this time I recognised that what I was feeling wasn't healthy, so I took myself off to the doctor and voiced my concerns. I most certainly do not want to get to the stage I was at before. (To be honest I don't think I'd have gone to the doctor had my lovely Admiral Nurse not recommended it). I have also found I am more willing to open up to my family about it. But opening up to the world is a different matter. It is so frustrating to be told to "just get over it" "think positive" "get out more" etc. etc. If only it was that easy, do you think I enjoy wallowing in my deepest darkest thoughts!?

The doctor put me forward for some counselling, and the office rang me a week later to organise it. After doing quite a simple number test (on a scale of 1-10 how frequently have you felt....) she analysed what sort of counselling I would need. She then informed me it will take up to SIX MONTHS to actually get me into counselling. Six months!?!?! Well thank goodness I have a good support network. Imagine the people who don't! Six months of spiraling further into depression with no help!

This led me to talk to others about their experiences and I found so many had similar problems. Frequently doctors are prescribing anti-depressants, when the problem that needs to be addressed could be done so through other approaches. For example a friend let me know about "The Linden Method". It is the technique she used to overcome her own issues. I have checked out the website, and although it seems expensive it tackles the way the mind works, rather than blocking it off like the medications do, which I personally believe can be more beneficial to long term recovery.

That is not to say I don't think people should take anti-depressants, it is of course down to the individual and what they find works. I have friends who find the counselling works better while using the anti-depressants, and I can see why. Sometimes you need to suppress the extreme feelings of negativity in order to tackle what is causing them. But personally I prefer not to rely on medication as I worry about becoming dependent. I have seen people who cannot function one day without anti-depressants, and it is not something I would want for my life.

To be fair to the NHS, I am still supportive of the GP's, nurses, paramedics and other staff members. I just find it unacceptable that people with life threatening (depression can lead to suicidal thoughts, which I think could be considered as life threatening) illnesses are being left for 6 months. The lady did inform me that there are changes being implemented in hopes to tackling the waiting list, but could not make promises.

Depression, as well as other mental illnesses, is not a weakness. It is not something we should feel ashamed to say we have coped/struggled with, are coping/struggling with. I feel ashamed that even in this day and age, people are made to feel weak if they have a mental illness. I am proud of myself, and others for tackling this massive obstacle in my/their lives, and I would not change anything about my past/present struggles with depression as it would make me a different person to the one I am today. And I'm kind of beginning to like her."

Writing this post was prompted after reading through the rest of my blog and realising that I had often mentioned that there was a cloud of doom following me, or a pit for me to fall into. But I hadn't really spoken in depth about why that was. It was hard initially to open up, as so many people still view mental illness as a weakness, but in the end that was what pushed me to writing so openly about my struggles. If we are going to make any progress tackling the public misperceptions of mental illnesses we need to be honest about them.

It still comes creeping, despite losing weight, despite getting my dream job, despite working on finishing everything I start. I think in a way it will always be there, trying to tell me I'm not good enough, that people don't want to be around me, that I could have done more, that things aren't worth trying for. Because depression isn't just feeling sad, there's a lethargy that comes too. A constant feeling like everything is too much effort, or not worth it, or doomed to fail. Things like brushing my teeth, smiling, or thinking. I become a zombie when I'm under the cloud, just auto piloting myself so I don't lose my step.

I'm lucky to have found people that can point out to me when I'm heading in the wrong direction, and that I'm becoming strong enough to notice it in myself. I've allowed myself to feel happy and I recognise when that feeling slides, which is OK, but when it starts to affect my wellbeing in any way I ask for help. And that's the point I really want to reiterate, asking for help in these situations isn't weak. Everybody needs support, and with the right care we can go on and achieve anything. We are only limited by our minds, and once the barriers are broken down, the dreams that we thought impossible can become reality.

Chapter 12:

December 2013

"Yesterday Nan and I felt extremely bored, what with waiting for Christmas to arrive and a storm brewing. So I thought we could play a board game. It makes a change from cards (which I am extremely fed up of losing). But I was unsure how Nan would cope, there's a lot of stages to board games and a lot to remember.

But you know what? There was no need to worry, or any reason to have delayed so long. Nan coped brilliantly. She said she's never played Monopoly before, I am unsure if that was true but she picked it up quick enough. Buying as many properties as she could hold. Then ending up in jail many times which she found hilarious.

Of course remembering what was going on and what she should do next was a small issue but a little nudge and she'd swing back. There was no problem with attention. We played for 4 hours, and I honestly think I got bored before she did.

Nan really loved counting the money. Especially when she had a lot of it. And she did such a brilliant job of giving me the exact amount that I barely bothered checking. The only thing that stumped her was when she had too much money, for example if she only had two 100M's and I needed 120M. The idea of change was something she couldn't consider, but that was the only time I really had to "take over" for her.

So please remember, don't hold someone back because you think they can't do it. Let them prove you wrong. Think Nan with Monopoly, and Finding Nemo with the swimming.

And of course to all of you, have a very Merry Christmas. From both me and Nan. I hope you take time out and can get in at least 5 minutes relaxation."

A recurring theme throughout my blog was Nanny Jean proving me wrong, time and time again. I was holding her back from doing things, thinking I was protecting her from upset if she failed. And then I'd relax and we'd do it together and we would both feel great after. To quote Finding Nemo "You think you can do these things, but you just can't"...And of course Marlin was wrong, Nemo could do it and so can Nanny Jean most of the time. And if she can't the world isn't going to end, she might become upset momentarily, but by using the techniques I learned along the way I can avoid her getting too miserable.

What if you get eaten by a shark: Acceptance

"Give me strength to accept the things I cannot change, the courage to change the things I can, and the wisdom to know the difference." – Unknown.

"Met up with a wonderful friend of mine for lunch today, and she inspired a new post. She is too damn brilliant. She knows exactly how I work, and knows more of what I'm thinking than I do. I wish I could do her words justice, as some of you need the pep talk she gave me today.

I have been fairly anxious lately, worried about getting a job, or going out and seeing friends. I worry too much about the what-if's. Her response? "What if you get eaten by a shark?" – My friend was terrified of open water, she worried about getting eaten by a shark, but she recently threw herself (literally) into a PADI course and is now a certified diver, and has seen things that she believes greatly outweigh the (slightly minimal) risk of being eaten by a shark. So why worry about the what--ifs? What if Nan has a fall when I go out? If she's going to fall, she will fall whether I am there or not. Hard as it is not to immediately shoulder the blame when something goes wrong, I cannot prevent everything. And going out will do me good, and make me a better caregiver at the end of the day.

So let's reiterate something I have covered before; "YOU ARE AMAZING". Full stop. My friend was trying to make me realise that I am a part of this. She told me (I'm still trying to get myself to accept it), that just getting through a week of what I do with Nan is amazing, let alone a year, and everything else I get on with in the meantime. You see, there aren't a lot of people like you and I that would give up so much to care for a loved one. Even if you don't live with an illness, you are still trying to do all you can. And that is amazing. And leads into my next point.

If you start struggling, and you have to stop caring and use outside help, or consider a residential care home, you haven't failed. According to my friend, I have a fear of failure. A fear that may have caused me to fail previous attempts at things by giving up hope before I had even started. Because if you don't try, you've automatically failed. But I (you) have tried, and I still am. And if there comes a day where the bad outweighs the good, it is OK to step back. No-one will judge me for not being able to cope anymore, but I have to be honest about when that time comes.

What about the guilt I feel? When I dream of all the things I think I'm missing? Am I going to mess up my future because I'm living with Nan (potential husbands will not be staying the night at my Nan's house!)? It is OK to feel guilty, but I (you/we) have to consider the things I want, and make time for them to happen. So my friend has given me homework (a 24 year old should not have homework coming in at all angles!), instead of a list of all the reasons why I'm amazing, a list of the things I want to have achieved by this time next year. And then she's going to help me figure out how to make them happen (I truly truly love this girl, the support she's given me throughout the years is insane, I would have given up on me by now, but she's still fighting away).

Another of my friend's points was to make more time for myself. Especially now I have started a job as a caregiver. She brought up my dreams of opening a drop in centre for carers like you and I. How can I encourage others to take time out if I refuse to do it myself? Much as I am already loving my new job, I do worry I may throw myself in too much. Luckily my boss is very understanding of our situation and I believe she will refuse to let me do anything that could detriment my own health, and Nan's. But I must remember it is OK, no, essential in order to be a good caregiver, to give yourself time to recover.

So remember; "give me strength to accept the things I cannot change, the courage to change the things I can, and the wisdom to know the difference". We cannot change everything, or prevent bad things from happening, but we can find the strength to deal with these situations. It may be hard sometimes but there are things we can do to change some situations, for the better. And it is important to know the things you can and can't control."

I'm a sucker for a good motto. I like to think they've helped shape me but in reality it's not necessarily the words, it's the way I've interpreted them and acted upon them. In this instance I was accepting being Nan's carer, using courage to change the negative outcomes, and when I remembered to be wise I acknowledged that there were times I wouldn't be able to change anything. Accepting a situation makes it much easier to cope with, and at the time I thought caring for Nan was my only option. I accepted that but didn't give myself a chance to view the other option. If and when I needed to I could let go of caring for Nan, I could do those things that I had left behind, and I was never trapped with Nan. I forced myself into a box by refusing to believe I deserved freedom, that once I had started being a carer that giving up on her would make me a failure.

But I did everything I could, and accepting I was no longer her best option is one of the hardest and best decisions I have made, for both of us.

Chapter 13:

January 2014

"Hello me again, nanny jean

had a bath today and it felt very good but dont think i have not washed because iiii always have a goodwash if i cannot get into the bath

kirsty told me it has been 20 years i cannot believe it. the demenshern seeme to have taken 20 or more years away asi cannot remember a thing about the last house i was in.ican remembe where i was achild"

"Nanny Jean is now eating her dinner but is finding it strange that 20 years have disappeared. She was stubbornly telling me the last time she had a bath was in a tin one in the last house. But when I asked her how old she is she knew she was 80 something. We have agreed that as the dementia has taken away 20 years it is only fair that she docks 20 years off her age. So Nanny Jean is now 60! I am so relieved that Nan let me help her wash her as I was becoming concerned about creases etc. maybe being neglected. It was relatively simple to get her to try it out, all I had to do was show her the new equipment. Told her she could try it with her clothes on, and then we slowly took off each item of clothing. By the time the bubbles had taken over the bathroom Nan was in her element.

"My bath made me feel lovely, I liked that it was nice. Relax into the bath. Yes"

So as you will all be aware Nan has joined the blogging scene, and the tweeting scene. I think we can safely say she has been progressing well. And she enjoyed taking part in another diverseAlz chat yesterday (write up to follow). I have noticed a few things beginning to slide again this week though. It's as if we can progress one thing, but we lose others, and it's a shame to think of what we might have to sacrifice.

For example, today Nan managed to sew on a button. I was pretty certain she wouldn't be able to see the needle and thread, let alone be able to coordinate the needle. But of course she proved me wrong, as she so often has a habit of doing. The button is securely back on her dress and she feels rather proud of herself. It may have taken her longer than it used to, but it is another thing she has achieved.

However, this week Nan has also been poorly. I won't go into details but it did bring to my attention more of a negligence in self-care than I was aware of previously. This led to some thinking outside the box, and yet another problem temporarily solved. Sometimes I feel like we are living in a submarine, which is being poked through with holes, and we only have so much gum to block up the holes. So we are just running around plugging gaps in the hopes of not drowning.

And here's one of our random quirks to think about, if anyone has a scientific reason for this I will be grateful; Nan can find her way around the house easier in the dark, with the doors shut than if the doors are open. If a door is open then Nan seems to blank it out, it's like it doesn't exist. So what is happening there?

And to end, a rather funny story of Nan's eagerness to feed the cat. She was unable to locate the cat food, so she improvised. What do you think we could feed the cat? Please, take some time to think a bit creatively about this. Ok, what were you thinking? Nope, it was shortbread. Poor cat had crumbled up shortbread. Unsurprisingly he was unimpressed and stalked off."

Nan still believes it is twenty years ago, or at least that she is twenty years younger. The concept of any sort of time really is lost on her, but thankfully she still has a regular enough routine that we have only had a couple of incidences where she has wanted to start her day at 3/4am.

We did try blogging again recently, after a long hiatus (while I worked at Disneyland). I'm not sure if it was being out of practice, or the development of the dementia but Nanny Jean struggled so much that I thought it was cruel to let her keep on. So I simply rearranged the format and conducted an interview (which was complicated enough as Nan is losing her ability to process questions and think of answers) which can be found in the last chapter as a guide to how far along Nanny Jean, Dementia Nan and I have progressed.

I'm fairly certain that even now with her diminished eyesight and lack of co-ordination that Nanny Jean would be able to sew a button on, probably better than any attempt I would make at it too. As soon as I mention to mum that I think Nan is unable to do such and such now she will completely surprise me and achieve things that surprise even the doctors (who have told us for at least the last 4 years to not expect her to make it to Christmas. We have tried to make every Christmas more special than the last every year for fear it will be her last. And here she is again, about to celebrate another)!

We never did figure out the root cause to the invisible doors, a few possibilities were bandied about on social media but there is nothing medical to suggest that people with dementia become blind to open doors. Obviously that was just a Nanny Jean quirk.

And the poor cat, he still gets anything Nanny Jean can get her hands on. I've taken to just filling his bowl with biscuits (which he hates) until it is meal time. So far the unusual cat meals have included; the shortbread, rice pudding, mashed potato, rice in plum sauce and many others. Thankfully between myself, mum and the carers he hasn't had much of a chance to sample any of these, not that I think he would want to.

Coping Mechanisms/Make 'em Laugh

"What with growing wisdom teeth, pampering Nanny Jean and taking her out to enjoy the sun I have been away from writing for a while, so apologies for the delay.

This was a post I wanted to write a couple of weeks ago but what with one thing and another it kept getting pushed back.

We all need coping mechanisms. I need mine for the smaller things. Such as when my Nan follows me round the house and hovers, just staring at whatever I'm doing. I like my space so this is probably the hardest part for me to cope with (apart from the central heating of course)! But I've found that explaining where I'm going, what I'm doing and keeping doors open to enable my nan to see me has helped to reduce the stalking. Obviously dementia affects memory, so another problem is conversation. We have been known to have the same three to four sentences on a loop for at least half an hour (weather is a particular favourite). I still find that I feel impolite when I change the subject but there are only so many times you can repeat yourself on a topic as mundane as the weather.

As you can probably guess from the title I have decided to write about coping mechanisms, for those with a loved one who is living with dementia. This was triggered by something you may or may not have seen. Rylan Clark (X Factor contestant) posted something on his Twitter, which made a joke out of a situation with his Nan who has dementia.

"Nannys climbed out the window down my aunts house..... Alzheimers, As sad as it is, you've still gotta laugh x #loveher."' (sic)

He added: "'Update! Nanny wants to come see her favourite grandson, she's on her way! Love her so much. Swear she's putting it on half the time x."'

For me personally the joke was clearly not offensive, but it caused outrage from many of his followers and ended up with him having to apologize. I also use humor to cope with my Nan's dementia, and so does my Nan. It is just easier to laugh about things that could cause massive upset to the people involved and it helps us keep plodding on with life. Should we be criticized for the way we deal with situations? Is humor the right way?

I believe it is the right way, as it helps everyone feel more relaxed, but there is a very fine line with using the humor as a coping mechanism and the humor being offensive.

Sometimes however even humor cannot help me cope, and I still find myself getting stressed, and trying desperately not to bash my head on the wall. Something I have found that helps when I get cross is crunching, be it dry cereal, carrots or ryvita. Crunching down on something hard repetitively for some reason really calms me. I mentioned it to the Admiral Nurse and she said that there have in fact been scientific studies that prove that crunching releases endorphins, so may even be something to consider to help Nan cope. (There's something new to try when you're at your wits end)

As a post note I would like to add that I also believe that sometimes my Nan must have "selective" memory! Sometimes it's as if she remembers the smallest things with no significance, but cannot remember the things she needs to remember. I obviously know she does not put it on, and it is a sad illness but at the same time it is amusing for me to think she's actually plotting against me, trying to make me insane!"

It still amazes me that so much outrage was caused by a comment that was obviously not meant maliciously. People spend too much time reading into things now, the glory of social media is that we can twist what has been written as there is no way to tell the implied emotion behind the type. It frustrates me that he backed down and apologised, why should he? Joking is clearly his way of coping, like so many of the people I have spoken with. Making light of the situation is by no means meant to harm or cause offence, simply makes it easier to process. And if Nanny Jean is happy to joke about her "barmy" situation then we should all take a leaf out of her book and enjoy life with a bit more humour.

I did mention the line though. There is a fine line between using comedy to cope, and comedy to offend. Any joke that makes light of dementia, or the people who live with it, I personally find offensive. The one off fly away jokes from the people who have no idea how hard it is to live with and adapt to. I tried to keep my blog light, by keeping in the humour that Nan and I live by, but it is important to remember why we are using that humour.

The crunching is a weird one, I find myself doing it out of habit now, when I'm nervous or bored. And much to my dentists chagrin I've started grinding my teeth, which I think may be from when there is nothing in the vicinity to crunch on, unless I want to chop up some concrete.

Other coping mechanisms I have used are waiting for Nanny Jean to go to bed and then spending at least two hours in the bath (repeatedly letting out some water then adding hot. Not that I advocate the waste of water). The problem now though is that Nan gets up every two hours to use the toilet so if I time it wrong I end up having to get out. I make sure I spend time listening to my own music, or watching my own TV shows. And of course I write about it. That was definitely my most effective coping mechanism, and always has been. I have about 50 notebooks from various points in my life where I've just needed to bear my soul. If I had any artistic talent I'd have liked to have drawn or painted my feelings.

I would say the best and safest way to get through challenging situations is to find a way to release everything felt internally to avoid self-combusting. I enjoyed archery, others kick boxing. Running. Screaming into a pillow. Find the thing that lets it all out, there are various more ideas on the internet which are definitely worth trying to avoid a buildup of stress.

To this day, one of my favourite things to do when Nan and I are having a bad day is to pretend she is putting it all on to drive me crazy. The dementia does seem selective at points so it is an easy enough thought. And because I am as stubborn as she can be I won't let her win the game, and it helps to slow me down and think of more rational ways to react to her behaviours.

Chapter 14:

February 2014

"As many of you will be aware, I have recently started working again. This was a decision that it took me a long time to make, I was so determined to be a full time carer to Nan, but it was just making me poorly. And constantly so cross. So now I am working part time and we have external carers in.

I didn't want carers in, it may not make sense, especially as we had them in Kent. But it took so long to find the carer that we both got on with and understood what we needed that I wasn't willing to go through all that aggro again. Plus in my eyes, we may as well have stayed in Kent if we were going to get new carers in. The reason we moved was for mum and my sister to be more involved, and granted they both see nan at least once a week now, but I think I was hoping for them to take more of the burden so we could keep it as family rather than strangers.

I agreed to meet with the social worker though, to see what we could get to help. And dammit she was lovely, and arranged for the care package to start 3 days after our meeting. Met the carers, and they were lovely too, and more than willing to help. They took on board what Nan said, and I felt comfortable enough to go out at the weekend. There was a mishap with the medication, but after one phone call that was all sorted. The care company here is already way above anything that I had expected. And so I'm feeling happier about having the extra support. Which is of course what they are here for.

In other news Diana is dead (does anyone remember our little plant we distilled the water for? She didn't make it), so we grew our own tulips instead as they are much easier to care for, and they are already sprouting. Nan feeling very proud, I just hope they get a bit more care than the cut flowers where the water went mouldy. I didn't even know water could get mouldy.

Nan is enjoying her baths, and is more than willing for me to help out. I had the less than glamorous task of wiping nans bottom yesterday, something which didn't faze either of us. And I think the fact that it didn't faze us made me feel a bit sadder about it, not so long ago Nan would not have even put her tights on in front of me.

When my sister asked what time I would be home from work my Nan replied "Oh I'm not sure, she goes all over the back and the fields..." and then proceeded to ask my sister what her plans were for Christmas (ten months to go!). I think this was my sister's first real experience of the dementia coming forward, as Nan has usually remained quite lucid around her. It seems the more comfortable Nan is with someone, the more the dementia shows itself.

And then there was Nan's trip out with mum, where she told mum she wouldn't remember her soon. Mum and I joked about this after, that we could pretend to be famous. But it hurts that Nan knows where she is going. We can all laugh and joke about it now, but I don't think we will be quite so nonchalant when it happens.

I'm not sure what's worse, the lucidity when she knows where the dementia will take her. Or the moments where the dementia is completely enveloping her and she doesn't know what she's doing."

Since writing this post we have changed the care group that were coming in, which is explained in more detail in the next part of the chapter. But we have been with the current company over a year now and with only a couple of minor mishaps. They listen to Nan, take on board what she wants, and what she needs. They treat her like a member of their family, and as jealous as this makes me feel sometimes, it is exactly what I wanted from a care company.

Yes I get jealous over other people getting my Nan's love and affection, but it is more than that too. Nanny Jean still seems to have enough control over the dementia that for at least two visits a day she will act like there is nothing "wrong" – to the point where we have had carers ask if we are sure she even has dementia. And like she always has done she is extra nice to anyone she doesn't feel like she knows, so they only ever get the nice Nanny Jean. Only mum, my sister and I have really witnessed the worst side of Dementia Nan, and for my mum and sister it was only recently opened up. I'm sure for years they thought I was overexaggerating.

I feel conflicted about the personal care, as much as I try to tell myself that it is a positive thing she is more relaxed which I hope is attributed to me. I know deep down that the dementia is just eating its way through her inhibitions. There are much fewer lucid moments now, so I'm really beginning to treasure them more, despite still feeling the worry. Especially when Nanny Jean gets that cheeky glint in her eyes, and causes as much mayhem as possible.

I think deep down she knows that naughty Nan is my favourite of her mood swings.

Candy from a Baby / Carer Conundrums:

"...I only wish today's post could be more positive, seeing as it is Easter. But Holidays don't seem to exist anymore, not for Nan anyway. So we carry on regardless.

Ripping off the elderly and infirm. It's an idea which should make most people's skin crawl, but unfortunately seems to happen with more regularity, especially if you scratch beneath the surface of companies.

I like to think that having me around, and my mum a phone call away means my nan has a little more protection than most, gives her a bit more of a voice than others. Unfortunately she has fallen victim to let's call them lesser hearted people, who robbed her on her doorstep. At the time this made me very cross, but the subject of today's post, maybe more so. Criminals and lesser hearted people, you would expect this sort of behaviour from, yes it is still wrong but I certainly find the idea easier to stomach than say a family member stealing from the elderly/infirm person, or perhaps the carer you entrusted?

Fortunately, in this respect the carers who have been coming in have not been stealing in the sense that they have taken money etc. from her purse. However I have been noting the times the carers have been coming for. And the findings surprised me. Say for example we pay them to come in for a half hour slot in the morning and a half hour slot in the evening. So you would assume I suppose that the carer would be in for an hour a day? Incorrect. We are lucky to have them in for an average of 40 minutes a day. Yesterday we had a grand total of 20 minutes visits from the carer. And the day before, no one turned up for the morning call, and only came for a 5 minute evening call. Over the period of one month I have discovered that we have paid the care company (who at this moment shall remain nameless) for 433 minutes of care that we have not received. The equivalent of just over 14 separate half hour calls!

How is this OK? If the company can do this to my Nan when they know I am here to oversee everything is shocking to me. Mostly because I know that my mother and I will fight this, but what about all the elderly and infirm people who have no one to voice their concerns? The people who completely rely on the care company? The ones who have become so ill that they no longer have a concept of time, and how long the carers spend "caring"? For how can a person receive the personalised care they deserve if the carers refuse to spend the allotted time with them?

I appreciate that there are now many people who require care, and that there is a certain amount of travel required between "clients", but why should each "client" lose out on time they are paying for, when surely it should be factored into the day of each carer?

I would appreciate any feedback on if anybody has come across this, especially if you have any ideas on what can be done to fight for those without a voice. Thank you once again to all my readers."

*   *   *

"Just a quick follow up to the previous post about the disappointment I have felt with the care company.

We have spoken to the boss and social services, both of whom have been very helpful and supportive, agreeing that travel time should not be included in the care time we pay for. They are endeavoring to ensure that carers coming to my nans house will stay for the time we pay for. I decided this was probably not the time to question the others who pay for the time but do not get it. But it is still something I feel passionately about, and I will be talking to the social worker in the near future as to what can be done for those without a voice.

Unfortunately we had more problems with one carer over the weekend, to the point where I have had to tell the company Nan and I have agreed we would rather she did not come to the house again. It is not that she is abusive or rude, but she has the wrong attitude for my Nan, and does not seem able to grasp the idea of dementia, or how to adapt conversation or requests in a way that a person with dementia can understand.

Which leads me to the question, am I asking too much from the carers? Are my expectations too high? I seem to get so much stress each week from the tiniest issues that arise from carers not doing things the way I expect, that I have considered stopping them coming at all. I know in the short term this will ease my stress, but I do not want to completely cut off the option of going out. Even though I refuse to go out at the moment as I am unable to trust the carers enough to have peace of mind leaving Nan alone with them."

Thanks to the dementia, Christmas and various other holidays and special events could well be any day of the year. My family have found this to work in our favour as I spend so much time in France, it means we can celebrate whenever we like, giving Nan multiple opportunities to celebrate.

When I was a professional carer we would not do any slots that were less than an hour. We found that even half hour slots are too hard to give a truly personalised and worthwhile experience. But unfortunately not everybody can afford the prices of hour long slots multiple times a day throughout the week.

As much as the social worker wanted to help she couldn't. I was essentially told there is nothing we can do for the people who can't fight their own battles. And she passed the blame to the government. I am trying to avoid becoming too political but there really needs to be more done about the care system. People are living longer, if we are going to fund the technology to encourage longer survival rates then we need to figure out a way for the survival to be enjoyable and worthwhile. Not letting people fall by the wayside because they are old.

I know for a fact that I was looking for issues, I still do. I still try to find problems that aren't there as it is difficult to admit that other people are able to things for Nan that I thought I was the only person able to do. Asking for the basics, like receiving the care that we pay for, that we have carers who understand dementia. That is not asking too much. That is asking for what is best for Nan, and what we deserve. Asking for carers who arrive at an exact time in order to keep Nan's routine, was asking too much and was me trying to find a way to keep some control over the situation, to still feel like I could help.

Chapter 15:

Respect Your Elders-Stigma

"I know I've been brought up well. There are some rules that should stick with you if you've been brought up properly. One of which is "Respect your elders". For my generation this is important not just out of of politeness but because our elders (grandparents) contributed to if not fought in the Wars. They are the reason we are not all speaking German, and that Judaism was not wiped out in the West in the 40's. Don't get me wrong, I believe to get respect you have to give respect (and some elderly people can be downright rude) but it doesn't hurt to be impossibly polite back and give them a reason to respect the younger generations.

So this blog is concerning my anger about the way that elderly people are being portrayed on the television. An episode of Emmerdale left me so cross today that I had to write to Ofcom to complain. And I threw in an email to number 10 for good measure, although I do not believe it will achieve anything.

Why is there still such a stigma surrounding elderly people? Especially those with memory issues? It's because people still aren't talking about it (like many mental illnesses. They are getting swept under the rug having depression blamed on phases, they'll grow out of it etc.). On the rare occasions when people are talking about it, it's in a derogatory manner. For example tonight's episode of Emmerdale "sitting like cabbages with soup dribbling down their chins". This sort of attitude is the reason that many elderly people do not wish to go into care homes & it hacks me off that people are so blasé in the way they talk about elderly people. Respect your elders? Also the incident I mentioned in a previous blog where a character in EastEnders referred to another character who was struggling with memory issues as having "lost her marbles".

I hope you agree this is unacceptable & something can be done by government to promote awareness of dementia and the effects on the families and sufferers. But for now, let's just get more people talking about it. I'm amazed that this blog has reached readers in America and Canada and Czech Republic! So let's spread the word further and ensure that this taboo subject gets tackled!

*   *   *

So this is something I've been thinking about a long time. Ever since I started caring, and became aware of what dementia really is and means I have been getting more and more wound up about the misconceptions I have encountered. So I asked around, and found I was not alone. And sadly, we rarely seem to argue or fight the people who are misconceptioning (yep, made up words. Just because I can).

I get so cross because sometimes I do argue back, but I'm thinking why should I have to justify myself? It's most likely none of these people's business. I should just tell them to get lost. But no, their judgements and wrong ideas sit and rot in my brain. Which doesn't help towards having a stable state of mind!

So what are some of the misconceptions that are encountered by (young) carers, people with dementia, families of those with dementia?

- *We found that people are being judged for how long they spend on their social media accounts. This makes me cross as Twitter is essentially my support network. I wouldn't be without them as they understand what I'm going through. So I can understand why so many of us feel physical/emotional attachments to our personal internet devices. It's our lifeline! The people on Twitter are always there for me, and I want to be there for them. That's part of why we get on so well because we stick by each other and never judge. If you want someone you can guarantee someone will be around to give advice, pick you up or make you laugh. I like knowing I'm a part of that.*
- *I struggle when people seem to think that I should be coping better because it's only my Nan. I haven't known her as long as say a life partner or parent and so can't be as attached. I try not to swear in this blog but you know what? Just **** off. I shouldn't have to explain my bond and closeness with my grandparents, and I shouldn't be made to feel that this is somehow inferior to the love for a parent or partner.*
- *Being judged for not putting a relative on medication – against said relative's choice. That because there is so much press about the miracle results, everyone should be put on medication. I think though if the individual, family and doctor agree that it would not be beneficial that we should not be having to explain. The misconception seems to be that if*

medicine works for one it will work for another, but of course we all know that's NOT true!.

- *I keep experiencing people treating me like a child, like I can't do proper care because she's only my nan and so I can't be suffering as much as if it was someone I had known for 50 years. Like I have it so easy and caring for nan is some cushy life I've chosen because I don't have to pay rent and if I want to stay in my pajamas I can, because I chose to care for nan I don't have a right to complain about it because I knew what I was doing. I have these feelings deep down anyway and I don't need people dragging them up to the surface. I know Nan is easier to care for than others. I'm lucky she sleeps in to 8 when other people are up all night, or have to be up at god knows what time of morning for work. But I am constantly thinking of Nan and her welfare from 8am till 11pm and I'm still thinking and worrying when I sleep. If I hear any sort of noise, I am up. So when I have time away, yes I sleep until 10 am, but it is a relatively worry free sleep and I feel like I need it.*
- *It makes me so cross when people act like some sort of expert when I have studied it (briefly), worked with it, cared for and lived with the by-effects of it, write about it, talk to people who care for and experience it first hand, and I KNOW I am hardly scraping the surface with my knowledge!*
- *The people that think there is just one sort of dementia and that those with it are selective about what they remember – I laugh about it with Nan sometimes that she will remember her ability to eat chocolate but for some reason vegetables are too hard...*

- *Companies who have a telephone script and despite explaining your mum has dementia they still fire twenty questions at her.*
- *Care company carers who are paid to come in and cook a meal and ask the client if she's eaten then leave without checking, she has dementia she doesn't remember!*
- *Mainly that people with dementia don't matter as they cannot remember anything anyway. Despicable."*

My message to number 10 didn't work, I never heard back from Ofcom or the prime minister.

I find it sad that we still use these terms when talking about dementia, the elderly or care homes, recent examples include "gormless" and "deranged". This is that fine line I was talking about in an earlier chapter, Nanny Jean is happy to joke about the dementia and its effects on her, but if I called her a cabbage she'd be rightly offended. I do have to give props to the entire Emmerdale team though, the current storyline following Ashley and his dementia has brought some much needed insight and coverage into what it is really like to live with.

As demonstrated from the second post, it wasn't only the misconceptions and stigma regarding dementia and elderly. I was struggling to fight people's judgements of myself, as a young carer. And the severity of my situation. It couldn't be as bad as other peoples.

I still get cross when people are judged for spending time on social media, or being on their phones. I agree there are times and places. And sometimes real life interaction is necessary, but at the time for me internet interaction was all I felt capable of. And for some people it is their only way to contact the outside world. Or the only way to speak to relatives and friends overseas. The people I kept in touch with online were my lifeline, they kept me, and Nan feeling like there were people out there who cared, who wanted us to keep plodding on. And I will always fight being told I spend too much time online for this reason.

I can feel myself getting worked up again just reading this. I remember being told on multiple occasions that because I wasn't as closely related to Nan that it wasn't my job to care for her. And that it wasn't as hard for me to deal with because I hadn't known her as long. And that I should be grateful I wasn't going through this with a parent. Of course, I am grateful that both of my parents were around, and were both of stable enough mind to be able to help me through this. But to diminish the way I feel about watching my Nan die (no matter how much I try to keep positive about living with dementia, at the end of the day it is still fatal) is unacceptable. Especially as I was living with and watching this happen 24 hours a day, making it kind of a full on intense experience.

The medication thing is still a regular question when people are told that Nanny Jean has dementia, which medication is she on? They all seem surprised to be told that she is not. And I've given up trying to explain to the do gooders and know it all's that multiple medical professionals agreed that there would be no point. That the risk of potential side effects would only be heightened when the medication is mixed with the cocktail of drugs Nan is currently on, far outweighing the possible benefits. That Nan is too far along for them to be likely to have any positive effect. That nobody, including Nan, sees a point in drawing out one stage of the dementia unnecessarily. I'm all for the medication being administered to those who want and or need it, but for Nan it would have been a waste of time, and I did not enjoy being made to feel like a bad person for being a part of the decision to not put her on pills.

Being treated like a child. I can understand that as teenagers we all resented it and thought we knew better and then we realised people were right and we didn't want to be adults yet, and being treated like a child is definitely best. But in the middle of my twenties I found it patronising to say the least that people were still acting like I couldn't know what I was talking about. That I would slip up with caring because I had never had any real responsibilities before.

That I was in fact leading the easy life because I could spend all day in my pajamas and not leave the house. That it wasn't a real job. Let me tell everybody right now, that some days being in pajamas all day just to have a bath a put a clean pair of pajamas on is the best. And if I have no plans to leave the house I don't think I should have to explain to anyone why I don't plan to make an effort. Nan loves my pajamas. Most of them are Disney themed so it gives her something to recognise and comment on. My lifestyle choices weren't affecting anyone at the end of the day. And if people really want to judge me for the clothes I wear while clearing diarrhea off of every surface then I'd like to see them giving being a full time carer a go. While looking immaculate of course. (Having worked in a nursery and cleaned up many nappy explosions I can honestly say there is a huge difference in adult and baby poop).

I feel like I could go on elaborating on all of these points, they all really get my back up. But I still have a huge issue with treating people who are living with dementia like they don't matter because they won't remember. That they don't need to be visited because they don't remember that any one has been. That it's ok to talk down to them or flip out because they won't remember the conversation. That their opinion doesn't matter because they'll forget or change their mind. Dementia isn't as simple as memory loss. It mixes memories, alters personalities and heightens moods, to name but a few effects. Nanny Jean may not remember that mum visits on average now two to three times a day but if mum doesn't show up one day Nanny will think she hasn't seen her for months.

Little things and effort make such a huge difference to people living with dementia, and to write them off is a waste of opportunity.

Chapter 16:

Fight for Your Right

"*Some may say I never needed more sass, some will say I did. But living with Nan is certainly increasing it tenfold. That and dying my hair red. I don't know if it's the stereotype, or possibly the chemicals in the dye but I certainly feel more empowered and fiery as a redhead.*

The topic of my hair colour does have some relevance to today's post. Which is once again nothing to do with any of the topics on my list. Just life keeps cropping up and throwing new obstacles at us which I feel I need to share.

A few weeks ago I called the pharmacy line to order Cephalexin for Nan. Had to make a point of which one was to be ordered as there is a brand that makes her poorly (shall spare you the details, it's enough I have to live through it). The lady said she could not guarantee it but would make a note on the system. That week we got the Cephalexin we ordered. Went down to collect again yesterday, and lo and behold they had the wrong one in again. Tried to send me home with it, and maybe the (meek-ha-ha) person I was a few months ago would have taken it and lived with the consequences. But no. Not today. I refuse to make Nan suffer any more than she has to. So I kicked up a teeny fuss. This is not the bottle she has. Half an hour it took me to convince the pharmacy that Nan is not just fussy, it's not the flavour she doesn't like, it makes her poorly. My Nan is not the sort of person who would complain about the flavour of a medicine. Grins and bears it. So after a minor tiff with the pharmacist he told me there was nothing he could do, but would order some in for me to collect tomorrow.

So today I went back to the pharmacy, and they made up the Cephalexin. Told me it was strawberry flavoured. Wonderful I said, but Nan doesn't care about flavour as long as it won't make her poorly. The pharmacist just looked at me (hindsight tells me it was a shifty look). Curious, I thought, they haven't given me the box. But no matter I shall take it home and try it. It is not our usual brand, but at least they haven't given us the one that makes her poorly. Or so I thought, when I got it home I noticed the label had a pink brand mark on it, suspiciously like the brand mark on the box of the one that makes her poorly.

Lo and behold, three doses later and Nan is poorly. And I AM LIVID!!!!!!!!!!

Nan now has to put up with being poorly until the pharmacist opens again Monday, and I can unleash my fury upon the halfwits. It's not as if she can miss the doses as the medicine keeps her kidneys working. But why should she be taking something that makes her feel worse, instead of better?

Why aren't the professionals listening to me? I live with her and care for her. I may not be a doctor but I know what she needs. Trying to fob me off with changing packaging is unacceptable. Trying to fob Nan off because you think she just doesn't like the flavour, when I have made it quite clear it makes her poorly is not professional.

Gods be with the people at the pharmacy Monday. I am sick of the elderly and ill people who get fobbed off and ignored because they cannot stand up for themselves. I am sick of being treated like a little girl who doesn't know any better. I am Kirsty, the carer and loving granddaughter and you will rue the day you acted against me. (Or something mighty like that). No longer will I squeak like a little mouse, my voice will be heard.

(You may be able to guess I have been reading Game of Thrones, battle speeches galore. Also empowered red-heads)

*   *   *

"A gentle breeze from Hushabye Mountain, softly blows over Lullabye Bay. It fills the sails of boats that are waiting, waiting to sail your worries away..." – Hushabye Mountain by the Sherman Brothers. From Chitty Chitty Bang Bang

Seem to be having a peaceful day today, which has given me plenty of opportunity to catch up with myself. Feel bad for Nan though, something is playing her up today so she's been silent nearly all day. She can't seem to decide if it's her back, neck, legs or ankles. I'd wager back but there's nothing I can do for the day to day aches and pains.

Today was Judgement Day for the pharmacy....And they delivered. Had to go through another round of questioning re: the flavour but once I had made quite clear the effects of the current meds he seemed more obliged to help. Did inform me that some antibiotics do cause similar side effects. Well I wasn't having that, I made it clear on Friday that we were previously prescribed meds that haven't disagreed with Nan, and I would prefer those. He told me there was nothing he could do. I explained (again) that Nan needs this med to keep her kidneys functioning so it's not something I can let her go without. He finally agreed to ring a colleague, who had another brand of the meds in but couldn't get them to the pharmacy til 4. Fine, I'll come back. Pharmacist did try to tell me I would need another prescription but I pretended I hadn't heard and walked off. Returned at 4, was given new meds, complete with box, and shown bottle inside to confirm it is a different med.

Nan currently taken 2 doses, and I have seen no side effects. So definitely stand up for yourself/your loved one if you know something is wrong. Do not let anyone tell you they are unable to help or change anything. We all know that's a load of bull, and if people really want to help they can. They just need a little encouragement. Which is sad really, I find myself expecting everyone to be as helpful and supportive as the lovely group on Twitter, or my Admiral Nurse, or social worker, or family/friends, sadly not always the case. But I'm fairly confident that the pharmacist will remember me, and what I'm there for from now on. I just feel a bit regretful I didn't get to use my battle speeches I had prepared.

Nan has reverted back to holding me tight, whenever I do the smallest things for her. And whispering that I can't leave. And that she's so grateful. But last night it was worse. Last night she told me she's sorry. (I started welling up). I asked her what she could be sorry for. "Because you're lumbered with me" Oh dear. Oh dear. Oh dear. Gave her a big squeeze, waited for my tears to sink back into my eye sockets and said I never feel lumbered, I feel lucky. Then ran upstairs to cry. (Hormonal mess, hay fever etc.).

It certainly is true some of the time. I do feel lucky to get so much time with my Nan. But yes, I admit it, sometimes I feel lumbered. What a horrible thing to admit, but it's out there. I'm now holding on to the thought that soon I'll be able to share responsibility with mum, easing her worry and my stress. Ultimately the message of today's post is in the title. Once again a lyric from a song. One of my favourites, Hushabye Mountain. Because at the end of the day, that's what I want Nan to know. That I'm here, regardless, to take any worries, troubles, and anxieties away and replace them with happiness, comfort and security.

Whatever it takes."

In hindsight I don't regret dying my hair red, despite being told it didn't suit me. I enjoyed it. And anything that helped me stand up for Nan has to be a good thing. And in turn I now stand up for myself a lot more.

I will go more in depth about the struggles that young people as carers encounter in the next chapter, as the issues I had with the pharmacist are just beginning to scratch the surface of people and professionals thinking that we couldn't possibly know what we're talking about because we have youthful faces.

Chapter 17:

Waking from tormented sleep/Guilt according to me:

"This is something that I covered in my blog, but it's not something you see talked about often. I suppose that despite all feeling guilty for one thing and another, we still feel ashamed of the things we feel guilty for.

I feel guilty whenever I leave Nan to meet up with friends, the what if's circle round. What if Nan falls? Or lets someone in? Or starts a fire?

And this in turn has led me to feel guilty about neglecting friends. And led to reluctance in me getting a job. Thankfully my friends have been understanding and I have a job where I can work hours around Nan. I've come to realise if she's going to fall, she will fall whether I am there or not. Hard as it is not to immediately shoulder the blame when something goes wrong, I cannot prevent everything. And going out will do me good, and make me a better caregiver at the end of the day.

I also feel guilty when leaving Nan with professional caregivers as I just don't think they can do it as well as me, they don't know her, not really. I feel so guilty if she is on her own as she must feel so bored and lonely.

I feel guilty when I get irritated at Dementia Nan's behaviours and repetitions, I know that it's part of the illness and I think that knowing that means I should be able to rise above it.

I dread the day I won't be able to cope anymore because despite what everyone says I will still feel as though I am letting Nan down.

I feel guilty about the things I might be missing, or have given up/will give up for Nan. I shouldn't regret losing these things due to all the things I've gained with Nan, and it was my decision to live this path.

But it's important to remember, and have people remind you, that just getting through a week of caring for a loved one is amazing let alone the months/years that some of us undertake. Surprisingly not everyone would. We are doing all we can, and even when it gets too much and we have to consider outside help, it is not a failure or anything to feel guilty about. We tried, and no one will judge us for taking that step away from the path."

Carers are constantly feeling guilty about something, it is the heavy burden that we all become accustomed to. Essentially questioning every action and thought as to whether it really is the best for our caree, or ourselves. And with the guilt of course comes the inevitable resentment, as soon as we start doubting ourselves our psyche kicks in and leads us to resent the things causing the doubts. It can be a merry go round of emotion in a carers head. And if not handled or processed correctly the guilt and resentment can build up and lead to detrimental effects for both the caregiver and caree.

In my time as a carer I had regular social media contact with other carers, and we were encouraged to open up about our guilt, to give it an outlet. And it turns out we all feel guilty for a majority of the same reasons:

* For worrying. We know our carees can pick up on our stress, and the fact that we are worried about them will only make them worry more.

* For not doing enough. Or for feeling like we could do more. The fact that we are not able to take it all away and cure it with a magic wand.

* For treating them like a child. Because we revert back to the skills we learned as parents and feel that by using these skills on an adult we are demeaning them.

* For feeling lonely. I don't want my Nan to know how isolated I feel, it's not her fault. But the way I approached caring led to me being very lonely for a long period of time. And I felt guilty that that feeling would be associated with her.

* Guilt for wondering about the future. Above all wondering about death for our loved ones, and if that would be a better route for them.

* Guilt for the resentment. Naturally as soon as I began to resent Dementia Nan I resented myself for feeling like that. Guilt can really mess with a person's head.

* Mostly though, we feel guilty when we give ourselves time. Time to relax, time to get away, time to wallow in self-pity.

So many of us feel guilty that one day we will have to ask for external help, that we will no longer be enough for our loved ones. And that's the one that most of us agreed deflates us most. That one day our loved one will need more than we can give.

Chapter 18:

Young Carers/we're the young

"We've got a situation, they're always putting us down
we are the generation, Can't keep us underground...We're on a one way mission, we can take it or die...Running the world, it's the time of our lives...We better start believing, before we run out of time. Fight til we fall, Standing tall...Coz we're the young, we're alright" (Mcfly: We're The Young, Motion in the Ocean)

"Great diverseAlz chat on Twitter today about young carers. Here's a write up and some added thoughts from me for those of you who couldn't make it (including the host who ended up in Twitter jail).

Our first question was how young is young? How can we define someone as a young carer? Aren't we all just as young as we feel? Guaranteed some days I feel older than Nan. Myself and another young carer are both in our twenties (she started caring for her granddad when she was 20! Astounding, I was still out at university, experimenting with life. And I don't think I would have been able to make a decision to care then). Which is apparently still outside of the norm for caring, particularly in the field of dementia.

I started off caring for Nan by accident really, I needed a place to live, and Nan needed some extra help after coming out of hospital with a broken wrist. And then I realised just how ill she was, and how terrifying the idea was of her being left alone. So I stayed, and a year later I can't ever imagine leaving.

We both found (as I imagine older carers do too) that personal care is the biggest hurdle. I think it's the role reversal that freaks me out so much. But you do just get used to it. It's really not something to worry about (and is, as my Admiral Nurse told me, a great way to prepare for children. Most carers have had their children and so know personal care inside out. Younger carers have it the other way round, and I think, once you've dealt with adult personal care, babies are a breeze).

The hardest part of dementia was something I think we can all agree on, when the one you love and care for, doesn't know you anymore. Or even just the confusion of a situation where they look at you so lost, and there's nothing you can say or do to help.

Another struggle younger carers are having to overcome is external attitudes. Some friends find it hard to accept that socialising with them is no longer a priority (this is why I am so truly grateful to all of you who stick around, because I feel I am not being the greatest friend I can. It is not that I do not care for you anymore because quite honestly I think of you all every day). Explaining to friends why you have taken on a 'responsibility' can be quite challenging, especially for me as I find it hard to articulate my thoughts when talking. Which is where my blog came in handy. I think some of my friends began to understand the thought processes behind me and my role as Nan's carer much better when they read my blog. And it's not only friends, professionals can be surprised to see a younger person accompanying a relative to the hospital etc. and quite often have voiced their surprise. Should we be having to explain ourselves?

I struggle to cope when I think of plans I had made, and dreams that I had. That have now been forgotten about, put away or quite simply refused. Because Nan, and the love I have for her, will always be my priority. But that doesn't make it any easier to see friends living the life I thought I'd have, happy couples walking around, or the books I have for travelling. In fact, honestly, it makes me quite bitter. The hardest question I was asked tonight was if I regret it. Sometimes, I do. I really do. I wish I could drop everything and drink til I pass out. I wish I could go window shopping, spend all day in bed with a fella, or loiter in the park (or whatever it is young people are doing nowadays). But then Nan smiles at me, or I'll remember a good moment. And the regret and the bitterness fades away, and all I can think about is Nan. Love comes first. And besides, even though I have/will have to turn down amazing opportunities, I have found even better ones in their place. Caring for Nan has closed some windows, but opened many doors in return. And besides, there is always the future. That's the great part of being such a young carer, I have the rest of my life to pursue my dreams. (And I certainly did that!)

Relaxing as a young carer is hard. Well again I suppose any carer. But all my friends are going out, seeing new things, doing the things I used to enjoy and I just don't feel I can leave nan long enough to truly enjoy myself. Whenever I leave the house I am checking my phone every 5 minutes in case there's an emergency. I am thinking about Nan and can't truly relax. (Very much looking forward to my holiday at Disneyland Paris. Disney is the only place I have ever really been able to switch off, and I'm hoping it can work its magic again). It was re-iterated once again though how important it is to have a break.

Is it really more challenging to be a young carer than a "grown up" carer? We were split. I don't think so, caring full stop is challenging, and why should my struggles be any worse just because I'm younger? The counter argument is that we are still finding ourselves, and our place in the world. This is where I worry, my place in the world is quite firmly by Nan's side. What about when she leaves? Have I set myself up too young? Will it be harder for me to find a new place when I am older? As I won't really know any different. I never set up a place anywhere else, I just wandered through life.

This chat made me grateful that Nan is not yet at the aggression stage of dementia (not sure I can rock the black eye look). That she is (pretty much) sleeping through the night. That my boss is so understanding and that my friends support me too."

While I was caring I couldn't see a life beyond Nan. I thought I would find it harder to find a purpose but I was very lucky to get the job I'd always dreamed of. I have to say working at the one place that has always been able to calm me has been a Godsend. And I've stopped worrying about the future so much. I'll have the occasional moment where I don't know where I'm going, what the plan for life is. But I'm so used to not having a plan that it works better for me to keep wandering. Discovering things I have passion for, that I'm good at. Keeping every option open. And that is what being young is about, discovery. At the end of the day I discovered I am a good carer, but that I will be much better at it when I've done the things I dream about. When I go back to caring I don't want to regret anything I didn't do.

The best way to cope with caring? Especially as a young carer? Educate yourself. Know what it is you're getting in to, how to get out, how to ask for a helping hand. Find an escapism. Bugger everyone who doesn't get it. And love yourself as much as the person you care for. You need time too.

Chapter 19:

Highlights/My favourite things

"What a day.

Woke up this morning, feeling almost refreshed. Scratched my legs bloody during the night but must have fallen asleep which was nice.

Got downstairs and Nan was fretting. She was sitting shaking her head saying "stupid" over and over and over. Made her a cup of tea and asked what was stupid. "Why can I never find anything?" Nothing I said made the tiniest bit of difference. Told her it happens to us all, asked her what she was looking for and she couldn't remember (which does of course make looking for it all that more tricky). But she spent the whole morning feeling sad, picked at her lunch and wouldn't talk to me.

Tried to distract her with various activities but she didn't want to get involved in anything. She was happy to watch me get on with everything but if I offered her anything to do she would shake her head sadly. This made me devastated. I hate the days I can't help. What can I do????? She wouldn't even watch TV.

In hindsight I've realised she was feeling like a failure, and wouldn't attempt anything new because she thought she would fail at that too :(. Had a few sad tears in my room.

Funnily enough she recovered in time for Deal or No Deal. And after she watched that she remembered she had been looking for the iron, as she wanted to iron the duvet cover. Apparently it looked creased and unattractive. For a lady who can't see carrots mixed in a casserole I'm amazed she could tell the cover hadn't been ironed. I told her not to worry as it would just get creased anyway. She told me she would do it tomorrow, on the bed.

So I went searching round the house, found the iron in the biscuit cupboard. Made an excuse as to why Nan wouldn't have seen it and took the cover off the bed. Nan asked what I was doing as I was getting the ironing board out. Why couldn't I just do it while it was on the bed? Because the duvet is not made for ironing and will catch fire. Over dramatised it slightly to emphasize that ironing things on the bed is not safe. Left a note for Nan to say I had borrowed the iron to do my work clothes and have now hidden the iron. As if I didn't have enough to worry about when I go out!

After Nan had cheered up I suggested we make some cards for mum to say thank you for our craft bits. Nan thought this was a lovely idea, so I got all the stuff out and she told me she had no idea what to do with it all. I asked if she ever did things like this at school. No, she told me, the war was on. I said well all you do is pick bits you like and make a picture or a pattern and stick it on with the glue.

After showing Nan how to work the glue we set to it, making our own cards. I watched Nan, and she thought very carefully about each shape, and colour making sure there was a pattern (not like mine, I am not very creative). I nearly cried happy tears right there at the table. She was constantly telling me how much she was enjoying doing it and held it up proudly at the end for my approval. I loved it so much

I had to give her a massive hug, and squeeze my tears out without her seeing. I asked her if she would like to write a note on it. She asked me who it was for, and once I said for my mum to say thank you, she scribbled down a lovely note. She even remembered that my mum is her daughter. Names and relationships are often hard for her to understand, so this made me even more chuffed. We have put the cards in an envelope for me to send tomorrow."

Even with the difficulties of the morning we still managed to turn everything round and had a great time. We kept the cards in the end. Mum saw them and was grateful but thought it would be better for us both to be able to see the achievements we made.

*   *   *

"Nan needed rather a lot of distraction today. Some blokes turned up to dig up her house (well really they were putting a new stopcock in, but if 3 blokes show up in your front garden with a pneumatic drill you panic, dementia only worsens that I should imagine).

I went and had a chat with the lads, they were very nice and reasonable when I asked about what they were doing so I could reassure Nan. Then I made them a cup of tea. When Nan saw me making the tea she calmed down. I guess in her mind she realised if I was making tea for them they couldn't be evil. But she was still clearly agitated. So out came the deck of cards, we went into a different room so she couldn't see them. And ten minutes later she was calm and laughing.

That may be because she absolutely thrashed me at cards today. I noticed a decline in her ability to grasp the rules, or stick to playing one game at once. We started with Rummy (she won 2-1). We played the memory game (not with the whole deck, just 1-5. She won 1-0). We then played Snap! And Beat Your Neighbour out of doors. I guess it's partly my fault for throwing so many games her way, should have stuck to one. But every time two cards with the same value showed up she snatched them. Every time she saw a card she wanted, she took it. If I tried to join in I wasn't allowed because I had to put some cards on her king. Needless to say she won whatever game that was hands down. Still, she enjoyed it. And I'm learning to not be such a bad loser."

I try to find any reason to not play cards now. I will play literally anything else in the hopes of winning. But of course because neither of us have any idea what rules we're playing by I lose every game we try. And I guess that's a good metaphor for living with dementia, no one knows what rules we're playing by, so just give up keeping score and have fun.

*   *   *

"We both woke up in such a glorious mood today, which after the tension of the last couple of days was just what we both needed. I had some cleaning to do so I put my music on, nice and loud (apologies to my neighbours). And Nan and I set about dusting and tidying, while singing along quite loudly to 'singing in the rain' (Nan gave a rather spectacular burst of energy to the line "and I'm ready for love" while I pretended to tap dance) and 'who

loves you'. As well as Nan's favourite 'Perhaps' and few songs from musicals.

Lovely morning and a great lunch time, Nan actually ate it all with no prompting. She spent a long time laughing, properly belly laughing after I told her the man who delivers it got his bald head stuck to the flypaper. She had tears in her eyes from laughing so much. Which is unusual, and so bloody brilliant to see. And then she helped me with the ironing. Well she folded and watched me iron. Then we decided to change the tune of the doorbell, and nan had a great time guessing what the tunes were meant to be, we settled for 'in the moonlight' (also known as memory from cats) until it gets closer to Christmas (nan said it is too early) and then we can have Jingle Bells.

We spent the afternoon doing a puzzle, which I thought would take us about an hour. It took us FIVE! Poor Nan was in charge of sorting the pieces, and she was great. Firstly into edges and middlays. Then into colours, then into how many holes and lumps. She told me she has had a lovely day, and I have to say so have I.

Almost as good as the day I had planned, watching Doctor Who. Which I am doing now while Nan dozes off."

All of the best days and memories I have had with Nan haven't come from spending loads of money, or putting too much thought in. They came from spontaneous moments where we both let go of our inhibitions and learned to embrace our quirky lives.

"Nanny Jean was happy when we went for dinner at the weekend for my little sister's birthday. I was expecting her to pass into the silence but she kept on top of conversation despite there being a group of 5 of us, she was laughing which was nice to see. She found it hilarious when another table moved due our raucous laughter. There was a nice moment after lunch when my mum told me that my staying with Nan had been having an effect. I'm not sure she meant this as a compliment however as she was referring to my Nan's new understanding of crude jokes and naughty words. But still, it's nice to know that other people can see the difference and I'm not imagining it to make myself feel better."

So just to prove to myself (and others who may be despairing) dementia doesn't have to make every day a struggle. Some of the best memories I will have of my Nan have come from caring for her, and I am definitely a better person. Not just because of the patience I've developed. But the confidence, and my willingness to be open to new possibilities. I would have been hard pushed to learn all of this in any other setting and I know myself better than ever before. I know more of my limits and am more willing to admit to them. Limits aren't weakness, we have limits to keep us strong.

Chapter 20:

Letting Go

"So it's been a while. Partly because I've gone off and got a job and a social life and just can't seem to find the time to write. And to be honest there's not all that much to write about. Nan's dementia is as ever present and steadily taking control of her mind but with no real notable changes to write about.

It's got to the point where Nan can no longer use the laptop, but she does still enjoy me reading out the comments and questions we receive. Nan is now confused most of the time, it can take the carers several attempts just to get Nan to brush her teeth, it's like as soon as she turns her back she forgets what she's been told. (If any of you watch doctor who, it's much like 'the order of the silence')

But it is no longer taking its toll on us and our relationship. Nan seems to be coping much better with living with it, and I am getting enough interaction outside that I can come home and not feel stressed or worried about what Nan is doing, or getting wound up by the smaller things. I may have taken things to the extreme but giving up caring for Nan was the best thing for both of us. In hindsight it was my pride that was getting in the way of realizing I should have done it sooner. Giving up caring felt like just full stop giving up, like I'd given up on Nan. But that wasn't the case, I was doing what was best for both of us as we were both suffering and becoming ill. And I was becoming overwhelmed with the attention nan and I were receiving, I've turned down so many interviews, and what could have been great *platforms to raise awareness because I wasn't ready, and that I regret.*

Yes it was hard initially, especially the aggravation of finding carers that suited both me and Nan that I felt I could trust. Hiccups are to be expected and of course it has not been plain sailing, but the ladies we have now are so great with Nan, and can work around the dementia. To the point where I can hear them make Nan laugh on nearly every visit.

And the time that I now spend with my Nan is much better, quality time, with my nanna. We still have our big chats setting the world to rights, she gives me advice on life and love. And is regularly telling me that other people's opinions shouldn't matter. So thanks to her, and the new friends I've made I'm learning to be more independent and to love myself and my life. Which brings me to my news...

Many of you know my love for Disney. Well I've been given a chance to follow that dream, and been offered a job at Disneyland Paris. It's something I've wanted since my first trip there almost 20 years ago, and it's a job I've been applying for, for nearly ten years. But this year is the first time I've succeeded and the first time I've felt ready. My life with Nan and Dementia Nan, and my recent new experiences with working have prepared me to move on to something I want to do."

*   *   *

October 2015

"It really has been a while since the last update! To be fair I think I have a good excuse for once. Regular followers will know I finally chased down that second star on the right and ended up in my own never land working at Disneyland Paris.

This may well be the last post about me and Nan, I'm shocked so many people still come back here and read old posts, and that the viewership is so high after being away so long. Nan and I could not be more grateful for all the support we have received, and I truly hope this blog carries on helping and educating any that need it. I will still be doing what I can raising awareness, and funds for dementia charities, because despite the boom in media coverage last year, many remain ignorant to the effects.

I think you all understand how nervous I was about actually pursuing my own dream and leaving Nan but as it turns out, we've both done okay. I'm back with Nan until my new contract starts at Disney and I don't think she even realised I haven't been here for 6 months. I'm trying not to disrupt her new routine too much as she seems to really rely on that now as a structure for every day but I think she's enjoying the added interactions.

For those of you who have me on Facebook there's a brilliant video of Nan playing the ukulele. She was keen to learn, for about five minutes. Then she took charge and did her own thing. As she should. As we all should, who gives a damn if it's not the right way? It made her smile, which is something I figure we all could do with more of.

Thanks once again to everyone who's helped us. We definitely wouldn't have made it without you!"

*   *   *

I thought it was only right that Nan got to update you all herself. Here goes!

"hello   helo my friend I my name is jeais jean i what is yoursdoi u amiwiiish"

I tried to get Nanny Jean to type up earlier today but it really stressed her out and as you can see, the results were a little muddled. So instead here is a little interview I conducted so Nanny Jean can keep you updated on her progress and feelings:

K: What's your name?

NJ: Jean.

K: How old are you?

NJ: Oh my goodness, fancy asking me that. I was born in January so I would have gone...no I can't remember. Is it eighty something?

K: Do you feel 86?

NJ: Sometimes yes. Very much so.

K: If it was up to you how old would you be?

NJ: I'd have said in my 80s. (If you could choose) oh, 50's (is that when you started enjoying life?) that is it yep.

K: Do you have a message for your fans on the blog?

NJ: Oh dear. Erm. I say hello to everybody and if anyone would like to give me a call sometime it would be nice and I'd like to thank them for keeping up with us.

K: What do you do on an average day?

NJ: Who me? Not a lot now unfortunately. I potter around, I try and help where I can but it's not very much. Dum de dump... talk to myself. Goodness me. I dunno. I can't remember a lot of what the time we did before. We did before. We did it before. Quite a while back. That's difficult because my memory is not like it was. I can't remember half the things we did. It still applies. (Can you remember today) *probably not. Things go out your mind.* (What are you thinking about right now) *nice cupper tea.* (What do you think about during the day?) *I try and find something to do. And sometimes I jot things to remind me.*

K: What is your favourite thing to do?

NJ: (Clucking noises) that's a hard one now.

K: Why's that?

NJ: Well it just is.

(Here we had a conversation about what a good answer that is and how my mum has the same answer – just because.)

NJ: So I take after mum, or she takes me then. I do like that. That's lovely. (Back to topic) *I like pottering around. And dusting.*

(Out the window?) *Traffic* (erm nope) *yeah I see Lorries* (think that's the old house, what's at the bottom of the hill) *well it must be a hill coz you go up it.* (So you can't see the ocean) *nope, never seen the ocean* (yes you can! Open the blind!) (Look out the window what can you see?) *Looks like rain.* (!!!) (Ok so. What can you see out the window) *traffic. See if anyone's coming.* (The sea?) *We're not near the sea.* (I gave up with this one after this.)

K: How do you feel the dementia is affecting your life?

NJ: Oh dear. (Big sigh) memories. It's difficult sometimes to remember some of the memories that I would have known. What else could it be? Going out, I can't go out on my own, coz it's dangerous apart from anything else. I miss going out on my own. Going down the shops which are not far away. It's trying to make top or tail of it if you know what I mean. I know I've got something wrong with me, or something that affects my brain or something like that so I take extra care when I go around or do things in case I mess it all up.

K: How is it affecting you personally?

NJ: Well I think it's slower that's a definite one. Can't keep up with how I used to be. It can be quite annoying, you think, you you know when you think what you've done in your past and now you can't do any of it or hardly any of it. (How does that make you feel) *awful – coz you're not what you was and you're not likely to gain it back.*

I have good days as well as bad days so it's not exactly erm sort of erm how do I put it no I don't know how to get to that one.

I'd like to say that I'm very happy here and appreciate what mum does and you do and Emily. (What about the followers?) *I hope that you all get good health or better health and that you're all happy and not worried about anything, people get sort of erm, what's the word to say erm. I dunno. If you haven't got somebody like you who helps things that I can't always get in my mind and I have to ask you and things that get I can put something down walk away and then forget where I've put it. Not really no* (worth worrying about) *you've got to try and put it aside and try and have a natural life not sort of bogged down."*

Publishing this book has really made me think about Nanny Jean and her progress. She has been living in a residential home for four months now, and although I've never seen her so sociable and happy, which is great, part of me is still sad. I am sad to see how muddled Nan has gotten, she can't tell the time, and she has no idea whether she's eaten, she can't chew hard foods, she often has mishaps with toileting, and she doesn't recognise any family members. It is nice to see her have positive moments, but it takes its toll on us to pretend everything is fine when we speak to her knowing that most of the time she doesn't register who we are.

There's so little of Nanny Jean left but she's still fighting to get through. But we both learned so much from each other, I don't think we ever realised how much we would gain. I never knew I needed her as much as I do, or how much I needed her input to turn my life around.

Check out my blogsite for handy hints, safety tips, exercises, activities, & memory box ideas:

Livingwithdementiablog.wordpress.com

**"Live Well, and Fight For What You Love"** – Nanny Jean 2014

For news on further books and other writings by Kirsty Elgar go to:

Kirstyfiction.wordpress.com

www.ingramcontent.com/pod-product-compliance
Lightning Source LLC
Chambersburg PA
CBHW050448290526
45786CB00006B/2210